10X The Kidney Friendly Diet

10X The Kidney Friendly Diet

Matthew Petchinsky

Apophis Enterprises LLC

10X The Kidney Friendly Diet
By: Matthew Petchinsky

Message from Author:

Hello, Reader!

I hope you enjoyed "The Kidney Friendly Diet", I am creating this book to expand more onto a full diet plan for the Kidney Friendly Diet. Take a deep dive into this book and keep being at your most optimal health.

-Matthew Petchinsky

Introduction to 10X The Kidney Friendly Diet

Rising Incidence of Kidney Problems

Kidney problems are becoming increasingly common worldwide, with approximately 37 million people in the United States alone affected by various kidney-related issues. These conditions range from recurrent kidney stones and urinary tract infections (UTIs) to more severe conditions such as chronic kidney disease and kidney cancer. This rising trend highlights the urgent need for effective strategies to prevent and manage kidney health issues.

Personal Experience with Kidney Issues

My journey with kidney problems began at a young age. At the age of 8 or 9, I experienced my first kidney infection. The pain and discomfort were intense, and it marked the beginning of a long struggle with kidney health. Not long after, I began experiencing recurrent urinary tract infections, which further complicated my condition. The frequent need for medical attention and the discomfort of these infections were a constant part of my childhood.

By the age of 10, I had my first encounter with kidney stones, a condition that would recur multiple times throughout my life. Kidney stones are hard deposits made of minerals and salts that form inside the kidneys. They can cause severe pain, often described as one of the most painful experiences one can endure. Over the years, I passed five kidney stones, each episode bringing excruciating pain and significant disruption to my daily life.

These personal experiences with kidney infections, UTIs, and kidney stones highlighted the importance of maintaining kidney health and led me to explore various dietary and lifestyle changes to improve my condition.

Emphasis on the Radical Nature of the Diet

The 10X The Kidney Friendly Diet is a radical approach designed to optimize kidney health through a combination of dietary modifications and lifestyle changes. This diet is inspired by the eating habits of our ancestors but tailored to address the unique challenges of modern life. The core principles of this diet include:

- **Elimination of Sugars and Preservative Foods:** Processed foods and sugars are known to contribute to kidney damage. This diet advocates for the complete removal of such items to prevent further harm and promote healing.
- **Incorporation of Alkaline Water and Reverse Osmosis Water:** Proper hydration is crucial for kidney health. The diet emphasizes the use of alkaline water to balance the body's pH levels and reverse osmosis water to remove harmful contaminants.
- **Focus on Meat and Alkaline Foods:** The diet primarily consists of high-quality meats and alkaline foods, which help reduce the burden on the kidneys and support overall health.

Benefits of the Diet for Weight Loss and Overall Health Improvement

One of the significant benefits of the 10X The Kidney Friendly Diet is its potential for weight loss and overall health improvement. While my weight has always been relatively low, averaging between 106-112 pounds, I noticed a marked improvement in my weight stability and overall well-being after adopting this diet. Key benefits include:

- **Weight Loss and Maintenance:** By eliminating sugars, preservatives, and processed foods, the diet helps shed excess weight and maintain a healthy body weight.
- **Improved Kidney Function:** The emphasis on alkaline water and a meat-based, alkaline food diet reduces the risk of kidney stones, infections, and other related issues.
- **Enhanced Energy Levels:** With a focus on nutrient-dense foods and proper hydration, the diet supports higher energy levels and better overall health.

In summary, the 10X The Kidney Friendly Diet is a comprehensive and radical approach to improving kidney health and overall well-being. By drawing on my personal experiences with kidney issues and incorporating principles from ancestral diets, this diet offers a promising solution for those looking to enhance their kidney function and lead a healthier life. The following chapters will provide a detailed exploration of the diet, its principles, and practical guidelines to help you achieve optimal kidney health.

Chapter 1: The Importance of Alkaline Water

Explanation of the Dangers of Regular Bottled Water and Its Additives

Many people assume that all bottled water is the same and that it inherently promotes good health. However, this assumption can be misleading. Regular bottled water, including popular brands such as Dasani, Aquafina, and Nestlé Pure Life, often contains additives that can be harmful, particularly to those with sensitive kidneys or existing kidney conditions.

1. **Magnesium Sulfate**: Often added to bottled water, magnesium sulfate is a chemical compound that can act as a laxative in high doses. It has been associated with neuromuscular toxicity, which can be particularly detrimental to individuals with compromised kidney function. Overconsumption of magnesium sulfate can lead to muscle weakness, lethargy, and in severe cases, toxicity.

2. **Potassium Chloride**: Another common additive, potassium chloride, is used to enhance the taste of water. However, excess potassium intake can be dangerous, especially for individuals with kidney disease. Hyperkalemia (high potassium levels in the blood) can cause serious health conditions, including heart arrhythmias and kidney failure.

3. **Low pH Levels**: Many bottled waters are slightly acidic, with pH levels below 7. This acidity can exacerbate kidney problems by stripping the body of essential minerals and electrolytes. Over time, consuming acidic water can lead to a state of acidosis, where the body's pH balance is disrupted, further stressing the kidneys.

Given these risks, it's crucial to be aware of the potential dangers associated with regular bottled water. For optimal kidney health, it is advisable to switch to water that supports the body's natural balance rather than disrupts it.

Benefits of Alkaline Water for Kidney Health

Alkaline water, characterized by its higher pH level (typically between 8 and 9), offers numerous benefits that can significantly improve kidney health and overall well-being. Here's why alkaline water is an essential component of the 10X The Kidney Friendly Diet:

1. **Restores Electrolyte Balance**: Alkaline water contains essential minerals such as calcium, potassium, and magnesium, which help maintain the body's electrolyte balance. This is particularly beneficial for kidney health as it supports optimal kidney function and helps in the filtration and excretion processes.

2. **Neutralizes Acidity**: One of the primary advantages of alkaline water is its ability to neutralize acidity in the body. By raising the body's pH levels, alkaline water helps prevent acidosis, a condition that can lead to kidney stones and other renal complications.

3. **Improves Hydration**: Alkaline water is believed to be more easily absorbed by the body, leading to better hydration. Proper hydration is crucial for kidney health as it aids in flushing out toxins and reduces the risk of kidney stones.

4. **Reduces Oxidative Stress**: Alkaline water has antioxidant properties that help neutralize free radicals, reducing oxidative stress on the kidneys. This protective effect can prevent cellular damage and support long-term kidney health.

5. **Supports Detoxification**: Enhanced hydration and improved pH balance aid the body's natural detoxification processes. By supporting the kidneys' role in filtering and excreting waste products, alkaline water can help maintain healthy kidney function and prevent infections.

Recommendations for Affordable Alkaline Water Brands

Transitioning to alkaline water doesn't have to be expensive or complicated. Here are some affordable and widely available brands that can be easily incorporated into your daily routine:

1. **Alkaline88**: Known for its smooth taste and high pH level, Alkaline88 water is infused with Himalayan minerals and electrolytes. It's available in various sizes, making it convenient for both home use and on-the-go hydration. You can find Alkaline88 at major retailers like Walmart and H-E-B, with prices typically ranging from $3.38 to $3.98 per gallon.

2. **Essentia Water**: Essentia is another popular brand that offers a pH of 9.5, ensuring optimal alkalinity. It's enhanced with a proprietary blend of electrolytes, making it a great choice for maintaining electrolyte balance. Essentia water is available in single-liter bottles, often priced under $2, and can be found at most grocery stores and supermarkets.

3. **Icelandic Glacial**: Sourced from the pristine springs of Iceland, this water has a naturally high pH level and is rich in minerals. Icelandic Glacial water is available in various sizes and is known for its purity and taste.

4. **Voss**: Voss offers alkaline water with a pH level around 8, packaged in elegant bottles. It's slightly more premium but provides excellent hydration and mineral content. Voss water is available in many supermarkets and health food stores.

5. **Alkaline Water 9.5+ Perfect Hydration**: This brand offers a pH of 9.5, ensuring excellent alkalinity for optimal kidney health. It is conveniently available at Walmart and is known for its high quality and affordability.

How to Incorporate Alkaline Water into Your Daily Routine

1. **Daily Consumption**: Aim to drink at least one to two gallons of alkaline water each day. This level of intake ensures that your body stays hydrated, your kidneys are supported, and toxins are efficiently flushed out.

2. **Consistency is Key**: Stick to a specific brand of alkaline water to maintain consistency in your electrolyte intake and pH balance. Switching brands frequently can disrupt this balance.

3. **Start Your Day with Alkaline Water**: Begin each morning with a glass of alkaline water to kickstart your hydration and set a positive tone for the day.

4. **Use Alkaline Water for Cooking**: Replace regular tap water with alkaline water for cooking, especially in dishes like soups and stews, to maintain the health benefits throughout your meals.

5. **Stay Prepared**: Keep a stock of alkaline water at home and carry a bottle with you when you're out and about. This ensures you always have access to kidney-friendly hydration.

By understanding the dangers of regular bottled water and embracing the benefits of alkaline water, you can make a significant positive impact on your kidney health. Alkaline water not only supports the kidneys but also enhances overall well-being, making it a cornerstone of the 10X The Kidney Friendly Diet.

Is this conversation helpful so far?

Chapter 2: Elimination of Sugars and Preservative Foods
Detailed List of Foods Containing Sugars and Preservatives That Must Be Avoided

For optimal kidney health, it is crucial to eliminate foods that contain sugars and preservatives from your diet. These substances can contribute to kidney damage and exacerbate existing kidney conditions. Below is a comprehensive list of foods that must be avoided:

1. **Sugary Snacks and Desserts**
   - Chocolates
   - Cookies
   - Cakes
   - Pies
   - Pastries
   - Candy
   - Ice cream
2. **Processed Foods**
   - Chips (potato chips, corn chips, tortilla chips)
   - Packaged popcorn
   - Pretzels
   - Instant noodles (e.g., ramen)
   - Frozen meals and snacks
3. **Beverages**
   - Sodas
   - Sports drinks
   - Sweetened teas
   - Fruit juices (apple, orange, grape, etc.)
   - Alcoholic beverages
4. **Canned Foods**
   - Canned beans
   - Canned soups

- Canned vegetables
- Canned fruits
- Canned meals (e.g., chili, stews)

5. **Condiments and Sauces**
   - Ketchup
   - BBQ sauce
   - Salad dressings
   - Pasta sauces
   - Marinades

6. **Bread and Bakery Products**
   - White bread
   - Whole wheat bread (contains preservatives)
   - Bagels
   - Muffins
   - Buns

7. **Dairy Products**
   - Milk
   - Cheese (most varieties)
   - Yogurt
   - Sour cream

8. **Breakfast Foods**
   - Cereals
   - Granola bars
   - Instant oatmeal
   - Pre-packaged breakfast sandwiches

9. **Processed Meats**
   - Sausages
   - Bacon (unless specifically sugar-free)
   - Deli meats
   - Hot dogs

10. **Miscellaneous**
    - Honey
    - Syrups

- ○ Jams and jellies
- ○ Nut butters with added sugars or preservatives

Explanation of How These Foods Harm the Kidneys and Overall Health

1. **Sugary Foods and Beverages**: Sugary foods and drinks lead to increased blood sugar levels, which can cause insulin resistance and type 2 diabetes, conditions that are closely linked to kidney disease. High sugar intake also leads to obesity, hypertension, and metabolic syndrome, all of which put extra strain on the kidneys.
2. **Preservatives**: Preservatives like sodium benzoate, nitrates, and sulfites are added to foods to extend their shelf life. However, these chemicals can be harmful to the kidneys, as they require additional effort from the kidneys to filter and excrete them. Over time, this extra burden can lead to kidney damage and decrease kidney function.
3. **Processed Foods**: Processed foods often contain high levels of sodium, artificial flavors, and trans fats. High sodium intake is linked to high blood pressure, a leading cause of chronic kidney disease. Trans fats and artificial additives can lead to inflammation and oxidative stress, which further damage the kidneys.
4. **Canned Foods**: Canned foods are typically high in sodium and often contain BPA (Bisphenol A), a chemical used in the lining of cans. BPA exposure has been linked to various health issues, including kidney problems. Additionally, the high sodium content can exacerbate hypertension and kidney damage.
5. **Condiments and Sauces**: These products often contain hidden sugars, sodium, and preservatives. Regular consumption can lead to an increase in blood pressure and blood sugar levels, both of which are detrimental to kidney health.
6. **Dairy Products**: Dairy contains lactose, which some individuals have difficulty digesting. Undigested lactose can cause digestive

issues and inflammation. Additionally, many dairy products contain added sugars and preservatives that can harm the kidneys.

Strategies for Coping with Sugar Cravings and Transitioning to a Sugar-Free Diet

1. **Gradual Reduction**: Start by gradually reducing your sugar intake instead of eliminating it all at once. This helps your body adjust and reduces withdrawal symptoms.
2. **Healthy Alternatives**: Replace sugary snacks with healthier options like fresh fruits (in moderation due to natural sugars), nuts, and seeds. Use natural sweeteners like stevia or monk fruit in place of sugar.
3. **Stay Hydrated**: Drink plenty of alkaline water throughout the day. Sometimes thirst is mistaken for hunger or sugar cravings. Staying hydrated can help reduce these cravings.
4. **Balanced Meals**: Ensure your meals are balanced with protein, healthy fats, and fiber. This helps keep you full for longer and stabilizes blood sugar levels, reducing the urge for sugary snacks.
5. **Mindful Eating**: Pay attention to your eating habits. Eat slowly and savor each bite. Mindful eating can help you recognize true hunger versus emotional cravings.
6. **Herbal Teas**: Incorporate herbal teas like ginger tea into your daily routine. Herbal teas can satisfy the need for something sweet and provide additional health benefits without adding sugar.
7. **Get Support**: Seek support from friends, family, or support groups. Sharing your journey with others can provide encouragement and accountability.
8. **Read Labels**: Become vigilant about reading food labels. Look for hidden sugars and preservatives, and choose products with minimal ingredients.

9. **Plan Ahead**: Plan your meals and snacks ahead of time to avoid reaching for sugary foods out of convenience. Prepare kidney-friendly snacks like cut vegetables, hummus, and boiled eggs.

10. **Exercise Regularly**: Physical activity can help reduce cravings and improve overall health. Exercise releases endorphins, which can help reduce the need for a sugar "high."

11. **Avoid Triggers**: Identify and avoid situations or foods that trigger your sugar cravings. For example, if you find that certain times of day or stress levels increase your cravings, plan healthy alternatives for those times.

12. **Keep a Journal**: Track your progress and feelings in a journal. Note any patterns in your cravings and how you managed them. This can help you identify strategies that work best for you.

Eliminating sugars and preservative foods from your diet is a significant step towards improving kidney health and overall well-being. By understanding the harmful effects of these foods and implementing strategies to cope with cravings, you can transition to a healthier, kidney-friendly diet with confidence and success.

Author's note:

Hello, everyone.

Now, as for the nuts, even natural sugars can trigger a urinary tract infection if your kidney is as weak as mine, since there is natural sugars or potassium. You can eat nuts but you have to keep a list of everything that limits your kidney.

I keep a list of restrictions for myself.

Keep your head up you will get through this. I am going to include a list section for you to keep tract of your food restrictions.

-Matthew Petchinsky

Food Restriction list:

1.

2.

3.

4.

5.

6.

7.

8.

9.

10.

11.

13.

14.

15.

16.

17.

18.

19.

20.

This is a rough list of stuff you have cut from your diet to help your health, especially dealing with weak kidneys.

Chapter 3: The Importance of Researching Nutrition Facts at Restaurants

Understanding the Hidden Dangers in Restaurant Foods

Dining out is a common part of modern life, but it poses significant challenges for those adhering to a kidney-friendly diet. Many restaurant foods contain hidden sugars and preservatives that can be detrimental to kidney health. Understanding these hidden dangers and knowing how to navigate restaurant menus is crucial for maintaining your dietary goals.

1. **Hidden Sugars in Restaurant Foods**:
    - **Condiments and Sauces**: Many sauces, dressings, and condiments are laden with added sugars. Ketchup, BBQ sauce, salad dressings, and marinades often contain high fructose corn syrup or other sweeteners.
    - **Beverages**: Sweetened drinks, including sodas, iced teas, lemonades, and alcoholic mixers, contribute significantly to sugar intake.
    - **Breads and Baked Goods**: Bread, buns, and pastries served at restaurants often contain added sugars to enhance flavor and extend shelf life.
    - **Desserts**: Obvious sources of sugar, desserts like cakes, cookies, and ice creams should be approached with caution.
2. **Preservatives and Additives**:
    - **Processed Meats**: Meats such as sausages, bacon, and deli meats often contain nitrates, sodium, and preservatives that can harm the kidneys.

- ◦ **Frozen and Pre-packaged Ingredients**: Restaurants frequently use frozen and pre-packaged foods that contain preservatives to maintain freshness and flavor.
- ◦ **Flavor Enhancers**: Additives like monosodium glutamate (MSG) are common in many restaurant dishes and can negatively impact kidney function.

Why Researching Nutrition Facts Is Essential

1. **Preventing Kidney Damage**: By understanding the nutritional content of restaurant foods, you can avoid ingredients that may harm your kidneys. This is particularly important for those with pre-existing kidney conditions.
2. **Managing Dietary Restrictions**: Researching nutrition facts helps you adhere to a kidney-friendly diet by making informed choices that align with your dietary restrictions.
3. **Avoiding Hidden Sugars and Preservatives**: Many seemingly healthy options may contain hidden sugars and preservatives. By checking nutrition facts, you can avoid these hidden dangers and make healthier choices.
4. **Maintaining Overall Health**: A diet high in sugars and preservatives not only affects kidney health but also contributes to other health issues such as diabetes, hypertension, and obesity. Researching nutrition facts helps in maintaining overall health and well-being.

How to Research Nutrition Facts Effectively

1. **Utilize Restaurant Websites:**
   - ◦ **Nutrition Information Sections**: Many restaurants provide detailed nutrition information on their websites. Look for sections dedicated to nutrition facts or menu items.

- **Downloadable Guides**: Some chains offer downloadable PDF guides with comprehensive nutritional data for all menu items.

2. **Use Nutrition Apps**:
   - **MyFitnessPal, Yazio, and Lose It!**: These apps allow you to search for restaurant dishes and view their nutritional content. They are useful tools for tracking your intake and making informed choices.
   - **Specialized Diet Apps**: Apps specifically designed for kidney health or other dietary needs can provide tailored recommendations.

3. **Direct Inquiries**:
   - **Ask the Staff**: Don't hesitate to ask restaurant staff for nutritional information or ingredient lists. They can often provide details on request.
   - **Custom Orders**: Request modifications to dishes to fit your dietary needs, such as removing sauces, asking for no added sugar, or choosing grilled over fried options.

4. **Look for Certifications and Labels**:
   - **Health-Conscious Restaurants**: Some restaurants specialize in health-conscious or dietary-specific menus and may offer dishes that are certified as low-sugar or free from preservatives.
   - **Kidney-Friendly Options**: Look for menu items or restaurants that specifically cater to kidney health.

Tips for Dining Out on a Kidney-Friendly Diet

1. **Plan Ahead**:
   - **Check Menus Online**: Before heading out, check the restaurant's menu online to identify potential options that fit your diet.

- **Call Ahead**: If the restaurant does not provide nutrition information online, call ahead and ask for details on their menu items.

2. **Be Cautious with "Healthy" Labels:**
   - **Scrutinize Healthy Claims**: Items labeled as "low-fat" or "gluten-free" may still contain high levels of sugar or preservatives. Always check the detailed nutrition facts.

3. **Choose Simple Dishes:**
   - **Opt for Grilled or Steamed**: Choose grilled or steamed dishes over fried or breaded options to reduce intake of unhealthy fats and preservatives.
   - **Avoid Complex Sauces**: Request sauces and dressings on the side, or opt for simpler seasoning like lemon juice, olive oil, or vinegar.

4. **Customize Your Order:**
   - **Ask for Ingredient Substitutions**: Substitute unhealthy ingredients with kidney-friendly alternatives, such as swapping fries for a side salad or steamed vegetables.
   - **Request No Added Sugar or Salt**: Specify that no extra sugar or salt be added to your dishes.

5. **Stay Hydrated with the Right Beverages:**
   - **Choose Water or Unsweetened Beverages**: Opt for water, preferably alkaline water if available, or unsweetened herbal teas. Avoid sugary drinks and sodas.

6. **Watch Portion Sizes:**
   - **Share Dishes**: Share larger portions with a friend or family member to avoid overeating and consuming excessive sugar or preservatives.
   - **Take Home Leftovers**: Consider taking half of your meal home to enjoy later, helping to manage portion sizes and intake.

Practical Examples of Researching Nutrition Facts

1. **Fast Food Chains:**
   - **McDonald's:** Check their website for detailed nutritional information. Opt for items like grilled chicken salads without dressing, and avoid sugary drinks and desserts.
   - **Subway:** Use their online nutrition calculator to build a sandwich that meets your dietary needs. Choose whole grain bread, lean proteins, and plenty of vegetables while avoiding sauces and sugary drinks.
2. **Sit-Down Restaurants:**
   - **Olive Garden:** Review their nutrition information guide to select dishes that fit your diet. Request sauces on the side and opt for grilled instead of fried options.
   - **Applebee's:** Use their online nutrition calculator to customize meals. Choose items from their lighter fare menu and avoid high-sugar cocktails and desserts.
3. **Ethnic Cuisine:**
   - **Chinese Restaurants:** Many dishes contain hidden sugars and high sodium levels. Opt for steamed dishes, request no added sugar, and avoid sauces like sweet and sour.
   - **Italian Restaurants:** Avoid pasta dishes with heavy, sugary sauces. Choose grilled meats and fish, and ask for vegetables without added sauce.

Conclusion

Researching nutrition facts at restaurants is a critical step in maintaining a kidney-friendly diet. By understanding the hidden sugars and preservatives in restaurant foods and making informed choices, you can protect your kidney health and overall well-being. Utilize online resources, ask questions, and customize your orders to fit your dietary needs. With careful planning and vigilance, dining out can be both enjoyable and healthy. This approach not only helps in managing kidney health but also contributes to long-term wellness and disease prevention.

Author's Note:

Hello,

Since I have been on The Kidney Friendly Diet, I find finding a restaurant to eat at is difficult for example, Mcdonald's had all beef patties, but the nuggets have sugar. Popeyes had tenders and nuggets without sugars, but the seed oils are a bit of an issue, but you can cheat on this diet with seed oils. Walmart has tenders without sugar.

My kidney has tried and tested a long list of places, but it does it upsetting for the restaurants to eat. Travel is difficult, you must check everything even with snacks.

-Matthew Petchinsky

Restaurants you can eat at:

1.

2.

3.

4.

5.

6.

7.

8.

9.

10.

11.

12.

13.

14.

15.

16.

17.

18.

19.

20.

Chapter 4: Mastering Nutrition Facts and Avoiding Sugars and Preservatives

The Importance of Reading Nutrition Labels

Understanding nutrition labels is essential for maintaining a kidney-friendly diet and overall health. Labels provide crucial information about the contents of food products, helping you make informed choices and avoid harmful ingredients such as added sugars, preservatives, and unhealthy fats. This chapter will guide you through the process of analyzing nutrition facts on all types of foods, including snacks, seafood packs, and more.

Key Components of Nutrition Labels

1. **Serving Size:**
   - The serving size is the first piece of information on the nutrition label. It indicates the amount of food that the nutritional information pertains to. Pay attention to this because it affects all the other values on the label.
   - **Importance**: Understanding serving size helps you control portions and calculate your actual intake of nutrients.

2. **Calories:**
   - This number indicates how much energy you get from one serving of the food. It's essential to monitor calorie intake to maintain a healthy weight.
   - **Importance**: For those with kidney issues, managing calorie intake can help prevent obesity, which is a risk factor for worsening kidney function.

3. **Macronutrients:**
   - **Total Fat:** Includes saturated fat, trans fat, and sometimes unsaturated fats. Look for foods low in saturated and trans fats.
     - **Importance**: High intake of saturated and trans fats can lead to heart disease and other health problems, which can strain the kidneys.

- **Cholesterol**: Found in animal products; high levels can contribute to heart disease.
    - **Importance**: Keeping cholesterol levels in check is crucial for overall cardiovascular health, which is linked to kidney health.
- **Sodium**: Essential for bodily functions, but excessive intake can lead to high blood pressure and kidney damage.
    - **Importance**: Those with kidney issues should aim for low-sodium options to prevent further complications.
- **Total Carbohydrates**: Includes dietary fiber, sugars, and sometimes added sugars.
    - **Importance**: Managing carbohydrate intake is vital for blood sugar control and preventing diabetes, which is a leading cause of kidney disease.
- **Protein**: Necessary for building and repairing tissues, but too much can strain the kidneys.
    - **Importance**: Balance protein intake to support kidney health without overburdening them.

4. **Micronutrients**:
- **Vitamins and Minerals**: Includes calcium, iron, potassium, and others. These are essential for various bodily functions.
    - **Importance**: Monitoring these helps ensure you are not getting too much or too little of essential nutrients, which can affect kidney function.

5. **Ingredients List**:
- This lists all the ingredients in the product in descending order by weight. Look out for hidden sugars, artificial additives, and preservatives.
    - **Importance**: Avoiding harmful ingredients can prevent kidney damage and support overall health.

How to Analyze Nutrition Labels for Specific Food Categories

1. **Snacks:**
   - **Chips and Crackers**: Look for low-sodium, whole grain options without added sugars or artificial flavors.
   - **Granola Bars**: Choose those with minimal added sugars and high fiber content. Avoid bars with artificial ingredients and preservatives.
   - **Nuts and Seeds**: Opt for unsalted, raw or dry-roasted varieties. Be cautious of flavored nuts that may contain added sugars and unhealthy fats.
   - **Dried Fruits**: Ensure they are free from added sugars and preservatives like sulfites.
2. **Seafood Packs:**
   - **Canned Fish (Tuna, Salmon, Sardines)**: Choose those packed in water without added salt. Be wary of flavored varieties that may contain added sugars and preservatives.
   - **Frozen Seafood**: Check for added sodium and preservatives. Aim for plain, unseasoned options.
   - **Smoked or Cured Fish**: These often contain high levels of sodium and nitrates. Look for low-sodium versions and consume in moderation.
3. **Dairy and Dairy Alternatives:**
   - **Milk and Yogurt**: Opt for plain, unsweetened versions. Be cautious of flavored options that contain high levels of added sugars.
   - **Cheese**: Look for varieties with no added sugars and lower sodium content. Avoid processed cheese products.
   - **Plant-Based Milks (Almond, Soy, Oat)**: Choose unsweetened versions without added preservatives or artificial flavors.
4. **Breads and Bakery Products:**

- **Bread**: Choose whole grain options with minimal ingredients. Avoid breads with added sugars, preservatives, and high sodium content.
- **Pastries and Muffins**: Generally high in sugars and unhealthy fats. If consuming, look for those made with whole grains and minimal added sugars.

5. **Condiments and Sauces:**
   - **Ketchup and BBQ Sauce**: High in added sugars. Opt for versions with no added sugars or make your own.
   - **Salad Dressings**: Choose those with simple ingredients, low in sugars, and healthy fats like olive oil.
   - **Soy Sauce and Teriyaki Sauce**: High in sodium. Use low-sodium versions and sparingly.

6. **Frozen and Pre-Packaged Meals:**
   - **Frozen Dinners**: Often high in sodium, sugars, and unhealthy fats. Choose options with whole ingredients and low sodium.
   - **Pre-Packaged Meals**: Check for added sugars and preservatives. Opt for those with whole foods and simple ingredients.

Avoidance of Sugars and Preservatives

1. **Recognizing Hidden Sugars:**
   - **Common Names for Sugars**: Ingredients like high fructose corn syrup, cane sugar, maltose, dextrose, and fruit juice concentrates are all forms of sugar. Learn to recognize these terms on labels.
   - **Naturally Occurring vs. Added Sugars**: Fruits and dairy naturally contain sugars. Focus on minimizing added sugars which are often listed separately on nutrition labels.

2. **Identifying Preservatives:**

- ◦ **Common Preservatives**: Sodium benzoate, potassium sorbate, nitrates, and sulfites are frequently used to extend shelf life but can have negative health effects.
  - ◦ **Artificial Additives**: Avoid products with artificial flavors, colors, and preservatives which are indicated by terms like "artificial flavor," "color added," or "preservative."

3. **Health Risks of Sugars and Preservatives**:
   - ◦ **Impact on Kidneys**: High sugar intake can lead to insulin resistance and diabetes, both of which are risk factors for kidney disease. Preservatives can strain the kidneys by requiring extra effort to filter and excrete these substances.
   - ◦ **Overall Health**: Excessive sugars contribute to obesity, heart disease, and metabolic syndrome. Preservatives can cause allergic reactions, digestive issues, and have been linked to cancer.

Strategies for Selecting Kidney-Friendly Foods

1. **Prioritize Whole Foods**: Whenever possible, choose whole, unprocessed foods. Fresh fruits, vegetables, lean meats, and whole grains are typically free from added sugars and preservatives.
2. **Cook at Home**: Preparing meals at home allows you to control the ingredients and avoid unwanted additives. Experiment with herbs and spices for flavor instead of relying on packaged sauces.
3. **Shop the Perimeter**: Grocery stores typically place fresh produce, meats, and dairy around the perimeter. Focus your shopping in these areas and avoid the center aisles where processed foods are often found.
4. **Use Online Resources**: Websites and apps like MyFitnessPal, Fooducate, and Yazio can help you analyze the nutritional content of foods and find healthier alternatives.
5. **Plan and Prepare**: Meal planning and preparation can help you avoid the temptation of convenient but unhealthy foods. Prepare

snacks and meals in advance to ensure you always have kidney-friendly options available.

6. **Stay Informed**: Food manufacturers can change ingredients, so regularly check labels even on products you frequently buy. Stay updated on the latest nutritional information and research related to kidney health.

Practical Examples of Reading Nutrition Labels

1. **Granola Bar**:
   - **Serving Size**: 1 bar (40g)
   - **Calories**: 200
   - **Total Fat**: 8g (Saturated Fat 1g, Trans Fat 0g)
   - **Sodium**: 150mg
   - **Total Carbohydrates**: 30g (Dietary Fiber 4g, Sugars 12g, Added Sugars 10g)
   - **Protein**: 5g
   - **Ingredients**: Rolled oats, honey, almonds, dried cranberries, sunflower oil, sea salt.
   - **Analysis**: High in added sugars. Look for a bar with less added sugar and more natural ingredients.
2. **Canned Tuna**:
   - **Serving Size**: 1 can (100g)
   - **Calories**: 90
   - **Total Fat**: 1g
   - **Sodium**: 300mg
   - **Total Carbohydrates**: 0g
   - **Protein**: 20g
   - **Ingredients**: Tuna, water, salt.
   - **Analysis**: Contains added salt. Opt for a low-sodium version.
3. **Bread**:
   - **Serving Size**: 1 slice (28g)

- ◦ **Calories**: 80
- ◦ **Total Fat**: 1g
- ◦ **Sodium**: 180mg
- ◦ **Total Carbohydrates**: 15g (Dietary Fiber 2g, Sugars 2g, Added Sugars 1g)
- ◦ **Protein**: 3g
- ◦ **Ingredients**: Whole wheat flour, water, honey, yeast, salt, molasses.
- ◦ **Analysis**: Contains added sugars. Look for bread with no added sugars and higher fiber content.

Conclusion

Mastering the skill of reading nutrition labels is essential for maintaining a kidney-friendly diet. By understanding the key components of nutrition labels and knowing what to look for, you can make informed choices that support your kidney health and overall well-being. Prioritize whole, unprocessed foods, cook at home whenever possible, and stay vigilant about the ingredients in packaged foods. With these strategies, you can confidently navigate the supermarket and ensure that every bite supports your journey to optimal health.

Author's note: There is sugar is in almost all foods, but you must be careful. You want a healthy kidney. Be careful what you choose.

-Matthew Petchinsky

Chapter 5: Optimal Meat Choices for Kidney Health
Importance of Incorporating Lean Meats to Avoid Acid Reflux
One of the critical aspects of maintaining a kidney-friendly diet is incorporating lean meats, such as 90%-96% ground beef, to avoid acid reflux and support overall kidney health. Acid reflux, also known as gastroesophageal reflux disease (GERD), occurs when stomach acid flows back into the esophagus, causing discomfort and potential damage. Consuming lean meats can help mitigate this issue by reducing the amount of fat in the diet, which is a common trigger for acid reflux.

1. **Benefits of Lean Meats:**
    - **Reduced Fat Content**: Lean meats like 90%-96% ground beef have lower fat content compared to fattier cuts. This helps prevent the relaxation of the lower esophageal sphincter (LES), which can lead to acid reflux.
    - **Better Digestion**: Lean meats are easier to digest, reducing the likelihood of stomach acid production and reflux.
    - **Nutrient-Dense**: Lean meats provide essential nutrients like protein, iron, and B vitamins without the excess fat, supporting muscle maintenance and overall health.

Detailed Guide on Selecting Kidney-Friendly Meats
Selecting the right types of meat is crucial for a kidney-friendly diet. Here's a detailed guide on choosing the best options:

1. **Beef:**
    - **90%-96% Ground Beef**: Opt for ground beef with 90%-96% lean content. It provides high-quality protein and essential nutrients while minimizing fat intake.

- **Steak Cuts**: Choose lean cuts such as sirloin, tenderloin, and flank steak. Trim any visible fat before cooking.
- **Roast Beef**: Opt for lean roast beef, ensuring it's free from added sodium and preservatives.

2. **Poultry**:

- **Chicken**: Choose skinless chicken breasts or thighs. Skinless chicken is lower in fat and easier on the digestive system. Roasting, grilling, or baking are healthier cooking methods.
- **Turkey**: Similar to chicken, opt for skinless turkey breast or lean ground turkey. Avoid processed turkey products like deli meats.
- **Duck and Goose**: These are higher in fat but can be consumed in moderation. Ensure they are cooked without additional fats or sauces.

3. **Fish and Seafood**:

- **Fatty Fish**: Salmon, mackerel, and trout are rich in omega-3 fatty acids, which have anti-inflammatory properties beneficial for kidney health. However, consume them in moderation due to their higher fat content.
- **Lean Fish**: Tilapia, cod, and haddock are excellent sources of lean protein. They are lower in fat and easy to digest.
- **Shellfish**: Shrimp, scallops, and crab can be included occasionally. Ensure they are fresh and not processed or breaded.

4. **Game Meats**:

- **Deer (Venison)**: Venison is very lean and high in protein, making it an excellent choice for a kidney-friendly diet. Ensure it is cooked thoroughly and consumed in moderation.
- **Rabbit**: Rabbit meat is lean and nutrient-dense. It's a good alternative to traditional meats, providing essential amino acids and minerals.

- **Bison**: Bison is lower in fat compared to beef and rich in nutrients. Choose lean cuts and cook using healthy methods like grilling or roasting.

5. **Lamb and Goat:**
   - **Lamb**: Opt for lean cuts such as loin chops and leg of lamb. Trim excess fat and cook using methods like grilling or baking to keep fat content low.
   - **Goat**: Goat meat is lean and nutritious. It's an excellent source of protein and minerals. Cook using slow-cooking methods to retain moisture and flavor.

Avoidance of Processed and Plant-Based Meats Due to Potential Kidney Harm

Processed meats and plant-based meat alternatives often contain ingredients that can be harmful to kidney health. Here's why it's important to avoid them:

1. **Processed Meats:**
   - **High Sodium Content**: Processed meats like sausages, bacon, and deli meats are high in sodium, which can exacerbate high blood pressure and worsen kidney function.
   - **Preservatives**: Nitrates and nitrites used in processed meats can form harmful compounds that increase the risk of kidney damage and other health issues.
   - **Unhealthy Fats**: Processed meats often contain high levels of saturated fats, contributing to heart disease and other complications that can strain the kidneys.
2. **Plant-Based Meats:**
   - **Additives and Preservatives**: Many plant-based meat alternatives contain additives and preservatives to enhance flavor and texture, which can be harmful to kidney health.

- **High Sodium**: These products often have high sodium levels to mimic the taste of real meat, which can be detrimental to those with kidney issues.
- **Potential Allergens**: Ingredients like soy and gluten used in plant-based meats can cause allergic reactions or digestive issues in some individuals.

Fresh Meat as Part of the Kidney-Friendly Diet

Incorporating fresh meat into your diet is essential for maintaining kidney health. Fresh meats are free from harmful additives and provide high-quality protein and essential nutrients. Here are some tips for incorporating fresh meat into your diet:

1. **Variety and Moderation**:
   - **Include Different Types**: Incorporate a variety of meats, such as beef, poultry, fish, lamb, and goat, to ensure a balanced intake of nutrients.
   - **Moderation is Key**: While meats are essential for protein, consuming them in moderation helps prevent overloading the kidneys with excess protein. Aim for balanced meals with appropriate portion sizes.
2. **Cooking Methods**:
   - **Healthy Cooking Techniques**: Use grilling, baking, roasting, and steaming as primary cooking methods to retain nutrients and minimize added fats.
   - **Avoid Frying**: Frying adds unnecessary fats and can create harmful compounds that stress the kidneys.
3. **Organ Meats**:
   - **Consume in Moderation**: Organ meats like liver and kidneys are nutrient-dense but should be consumed in moderation due to their high cholesterol content.

- Digestive Considerations: Individual tolerance varies, so monitor how your digestive system responds to organ meats and adjust your intake accordingly.

Practical Examples and Recipes

1. **Grilled Chicken Breast with Herbs:**
   - **Ingredients**: Skinless chicken breasts, olive oil, garlic, rosemary, thyme, salt, and pepper.
   - **Instructions**: Marinate chicken in olive oil, garlic, and herbs. Grill until fully cooked. Serve with steamed vegetables.
2. **Baked Salmon with Lemon and Dill:**
   - **Ingredients**: Salmon fillets, lemon slices, fresh dill, olive oil, salt, and pepper.
   - **Instructions**: Place salmon fillets on a baking sheet. Drizzle with olive oil, top with lemon slices and dill. Bake at 375°F (190°C) for 20-25 minutes.
3. **Venison Stew:**
   - **Ingredients**: Venison chunks, carrots, potatoes, onions, garlic, beef broth, salt, and pepper.
   - **Instructions**: Brown venison in a pot with olive oil. Add vegetables and broth. Simmer until meat and vegetables are tender. Season to taste.

Conclusion

Choosing the right meats is a crucial aspect of maintaining a kidney-friendly diet. By incorporating lean meats like 90%-96% ground beef, chicken, turkey, and various game meats, you can provide your body with essential nutrients while avoiding potential triggers for acid reflux and kidney damage. Avoid processed and plant-based meats due to their high sodium content and harmful additives. Embrace fresh meats, cooked using healthy methods, to support your kidney health and overall well-being. With careful selection and preparation, you can enjoy a varied and satisfying diet that promotes long-term health.

Chapter 6: Alkaline Foods for Kidney Health
The Importance of Alkaline Foods for Kidney Health

Alkaline foods play a vital role in supporting kidney function and overall health by helping to balance the body's pH levels, reducing acid load, and providing essential nutrients. A diet rich in alkaline foods, combined with lean meats, can improve kidney function, reduce inflammation, and promote general well-being. This chapter will provide a comprehensive list of alkaline foods, daily meal plans incorporating these foods, and the benefits of a predominantly meat and alkaline foods diet.

List of Alkaline Foods That Support Kidney Function and Overall Health

1. **Vegetables:**
   - **Leafy Greens**: Spinach, kale, Swiss chard, and collard greens.
   - **Cruciferous Vegetables**: Broccoli, cauliflower, Brussels sprouts, and cabbage.
   - **Root Vegetables**: Carrots, beets, sweet potatoes, and radishes.
   - **Other Vegetables**: Cucumbers, zucchini, bell peppers, and celery.
2. **Fruits** (in moderation due to natural sugars):
   - **Berries**: Strawberries, blueberries, raspberries, and blackberries.
   - **Citrus Fruits**: Lemons, limes, and grapefruits.
   - **Other Fruits**: Apples, pears, peaches, and cherries.
3. **Nuts and Seeds:**
   - **Almonds**
   - **Chia Seeds**

- Flaxseeds
- Pumpkin Seeds
4. **Legumes** (in moderation):
    - Lentils
    - Chickpeas
    - Black Beans
    - Kidney Beans
5. **Herbs and Spices:**
    - Basil
    - Parsley
    - Cilantro
    - Garlic
    - Ginger
6. **Healthy Fats:**
    - Avocados
    - Olive Oil
    - Coconut Oil
7. **Other Alkaline Foods:**
    - Quinoa
    - Buckwheat
    - Millet
8. **Onions:** Onions are particularly beneficial as they pair well with meats and enhance the flavor of various dishes. They are also rich in antioxidants and can help reduce inflammation.

Examples of Daily Meal Plans Incorporating Alkaline Foods

Here are some examples of daily meal plans that incorporate alkaline foods along with lean meats to support kidney health:

Day 1:

- **Breakfast:**
    - Scrambled eggs with spinach and cherry tomatoes
    - A small bowl of mixed berries

- ◦ Herbal tea (e.g., ginger tea)
- **Lunch:**
  - ◦ Grilled chicken breast with a side salad (mixed greens, cucumbers, bell peppers, and avocado) dressed with olive oil and lemon juice
  - ◦ A serving of quinoa
- **Snack:**
  - ◦ Sliced apple with a handful of almonds
- **Dinner:**
  - ◦ Baked salmon with roasted broccoli and sweet potatoes
  - ◦ A side of sautéed onions and garlic

Day 2:

- **Breakfast:**
  - ◦ Smoothie with kale, cucumber, lemon, chia seeds, and a small piece of fruit (e.g., apple)
  - ◦ A handful of walnuts
- **Lunch:**
  - ◦ Turkey and avocado wrap using a whole grain tortilla, filled with leafy greens and sliced onions
  - ◦ Carrot sticks with hummus
- **Snack:**
  - ◦ A small bowl of mixed berries
- **Dinner:**
  - ◦ Grilled lamb chops with a side of roasted Brussels sprouts and radishes
  - ◦ A serving of millet with sautéed onions and garlic

Day 3:

- **Breakfast:**

- Greek yogurt (plain, unsweetened) with a sprinkle of flax-seeds and a few raspberries
  - Herbal tea (e.g., peppermint tea)
- **Lunch:**
  - Salad with mixed greens, beets, avocado, chickpeas, and a lemon-tahini dressing
  - A serving of buckwheat
- **Snack:**
  - Celery sticks with almond butter
- **Dinner:**
  - Roasted chicken thighs with a side of sautéed kale and garlic
  - A side of quinoa with diced onions and parsley

Benefits of a Predominantly Meat and Alkaline Foods Diet

1. **Balanced pH Levels:**
   - Alkaline foods help neutralize excess acid in the body, promoting a balanced pH level. This balance is crucial for optimal kidney function as it reduces the workload on the kidneys to maintain the body's acid-base balance.
2. **Reduced Inflammation:**
   - Many alkaline foods, such as leafy greens, berries, and nuts, have anti-inflammatory properties. Reducing inflammation helps protect the kidneys from damage and supports overall health.
3. **Improved Kidney Function:**
   - A diet rich in alkaline foods and lean meats provides essential nutrients that support kidney function. These nutrients include antioxidants, vitamins, and minerals that help maintain healthy kidney tissue and function.
4. **Enhanced Digestion:**
   - Alkaline foods can improve digestive health by promoting a healthy gut microbiome and aiding in the digestion of

proteins and fats from meats. This synergy helps reduce digestive discomfort and supports nutrient absorption.

5. **Weight Management:**
   - Alkaline foods are typically low in calories and high in nutrients, which can help with weight management. Maintaining a healthy weight reduces the risk of developing kidney-related issues and other chronic diseases.

6. **Cardiovascular Health:**
   - The combination of lean meats and alkaline foods supports cardiovascular health by providing healthy fats, fiber, and antioxidants. This reduces the risk of hypertension and cardiovascular disease, which are closely linked to kidney health.

7. **Sustained Energy Levels:**
   - Alkaline foods provide a steady release of energy, helping to maintain stable blood sugar levels. Combined with the high-quality protein from lean meats, this diet ensures sustained energy levels throughout the day.

8. **Improved Immune Function:**
   - The nutrients found in alkaline foods, such as vitamins C and E, zinc, and selenium, support a robust immune system. A strong immune system helps protect against infections that can harm the kidneys.

Practical Tips for Incorporating Alkaline Foods and Meats into Your Diet

1. **Meal Planning:**
   - Plan your meals ahead of time to ensure a balanced intake of alkaline foods and lean meats. Preparing meals in advance can help you stick to your diet and avoid unhealthy options.

2. **Cooking Methods:**

- Use healthy cooking methods such as grilling, baking, steaming, and sautéing with minimal oil. Avoid frying and heavy sauces that can add unnecessary fats and calories.

3. **Fresh Ingredients:**
    - Choose fresh, whole ingredients whenever possible. Fresh vegetables, fruits, and meats provide the highest nutrient content and the best health benefits.

4. **Herbs and Spices:**
    - Enhance the flavor of your meals with herbs and spices instead of relying on salt and sugar. Herbs like parsley, cilantro, and basil, and spices like garlic and ginger, add flavor and health benefits.

5. **Moderation:**
    - While lean meats and alkaline foods are beneficial, moderation is key. Balance your intake to ensure you are getting a variety of nutrients from different sources.

6. **Listen to Your Body:**
    - Pay attention to how your body responds to different foods. Adjust your diet based on how you feel, and consult with a healthcare professional if you have specific health concerns or dietary needs.

Conclusion

Incorporating alkaline foods and lean meats into your diet is essential for supporting kidney health and overall well-being. By choosing the right foods and preparing them in a healthy manner, you can create delicious, nutrient-rich meals that promote optimal kidney function, reduce inflammation, and enhance your overall health. Embrace the benefits of a predominantly meat and alkaline foods diet and take proactive steps towards a healthier, more balanced lifestyle.

Chapter 7: Avoid Acidic Foods for Kidney Health

Understanding the Impact of Acidic Foods on Kidney Health

Acidic foods can pose significant challenges for individuals with weak or compromised kidneys. These foods increase the acid load in the body, which can exacerbate kidney problems and lead to conditions such as urinary tract infections (UTIs) and kidney stones. This chapter will provide an in-depth look at why it's essential to avoid acidic foods, a list of common acidic foods to avoid, and strategies for maintaining a balanced, kidney-friendly diet.

Why Avoiding Acidic Foods is Crucial for Kidney Health

1. **Increased Acid Load:**
   - **Acidosis**: Consuming acidic foods can lead to acidosis, a condition where there is too much acid in the body fluids. The kidneys must work harder to maintain the body's pH balance, which can further stress already weak kidneys.
   - **Kidney Strain**: Acidic foods increase the burden on the kidneys to filter and excrete excess acids, potentially worsening kidney function over time.

2. **Risk of Urinary Tract Infections (UTIs):**
   - **Irritation of Urinary Tract**: Acidic foods can irritate the urinary tract lining, making it more susceptible to infections. This is particularly problematic for individuals with compromised kidney function.
   - **Alkaline Balance**: Maintaining an alkaline balance in the body helps create an environment less conducive to bacterial growth, thereby reducing the risk of UTIs.

3. **Formation of Kidney Stones:**
   - **Oxalates and Uric Acid**: Certain acidic foods are high in oxalates and uric acid, which can contribute to the

formation of kidney stones. Avoiding these foods can help prevent the recurrence of stones.

List of Common Acidic Foods to Avoid

1. **Fruits:**
   - **Tomatoes**: Highly acidic and can exacerbate symptoms in individuals with weak kidneys.
   - **Blueberries**: Despite their health benefits, they are acidic and can irritate the urinary tract.
   - **Citrus Fruits**: Oranges, lemons, limes, and grapefruits are highly acidic and should be consumed in moderation.
   - **Pineapples**: Another fruit high in acid that can irritate the urinary system.

2. **Vegetables:**
   - **Tomatoes and Tomato Products**: Including tomato sauce, paste, and ketchup.
   - **Peppers**: While bell peppers are less acidic, hot peppers can contribute to acidity.
   - **Onions**: Although onions have many health benefits, they can be acidic for some individuals and should be consumed in moderation if they cause discomfort.

3. **Dairy Products:**
   - **Cheese**: Many types of cheese, especially aged varieties, are acidic.
   - **Yogurt**: While generally considered healthy, yogurt can be acidic, especially when sweetened.

4. **Grains and Processed Foods:**
   - **White Bread**: Highly processed and can be acidic.
   - **Pasta**: Particularly when made with refined grains.
   - **Processed Snacks**: Chips, crackers, and other processed snacks often have added preservatives and acids.

5. **Beverages:**

- **Sodas**: Highly acidic and should be avoided entirely.
- **Alcohol**: Especially beer and wine, which can increase acidity.
- **Coffee**: Acidic and can be harsh on the kidneys and urinary tract.

6. **Proteins:**
   - **Processed Meats**: Sausages, hot dogs, and deli meats are not only high in sodium but also acidic.
   - **Red Meat**: While not inherently acidic, red meat can increase acid production in the body and should be consumed in moderation.

Strategies for Maintaining a Balanced, Kidney-Friendly Diet

1. **Focus on Alkaline Foods:**
   - **Vegetables**: Leafy greens, cucumbers, bell peppers, and zucchini are all alkaline and beneficial for kidney health.
   - **Fruits**: Opt for low-acid fruits like apples, pears, and melons.
   - **Herbs and Spices**: Use herbs like basil, parsley, and cilantro to flavor your food instead of acidic condiments.
2. **Incorporate Lean Proteins:**
   - **Chicken and Turkey**: These are less likely to increase acidity and are excellent sources of lean protein.
   - **Fish**: Preferable to red meat, fish like salmon and trout also provide beneficial omega-3 fatty acids.
   - **Legumes**: Beans and lentils are good protein sources and generally less acidic.
3. **Hydration:**
   - **Alkaline Water**: Drinking alkaline water can help neutralize body acids and support kidney function.

- ◦ **Herbal Teas**: Ginger tea, peppermint tea, and other herbal teas are good alternatives to acidic beverages like coffee and soda.

4. **Meal Planning**:
   - ◦ **Balanced Meals**: Ensure each meal includes a good portion of alkaline vegetables, lean protein, and a moderate amount of whole grains.
   - ◦ **Avoid Processed Foods**: Stick to whole, natural foods as much as possible to avoid hidden acids and preservatives.

5. **Cooking Methods**:
   - ◦ **Avoid Frying**: Frying can increase the acidity of foods. Opt for grilling, baking, steaming, or roasting.
   - ◦ **Use Fresh Ingredients**: Fresh, organic produce and meats are less likely to contain additives that can increase acidity.

Practical Examples of Acidic Food Substitutions

1. **Instead of Tomatoes**:
   - ◦ **Use Red Bell Peppers**: They can provide a similar color and texture in dishes without the acidity.
   - ◦ **Make Pesto Sauce**: A basil pesto sauce can be a great alternative to tomato-based sauces.

2. **Instead of Blueberries**:
   - ◦ **Use Strawberries or Blackberries**: They are lower in acid and still provide a burst of flavor and antioxidants.
   - ◦ **Add Melons to Salads**: Melons like cantaloupe and honeydew are refreshing and low in acid.

3. **Instead of Citrus Fruits**:
   - ◦ **Choose Apples and Pears**: These fruits are lower in acid and versatile for snacking and cooking.
   - ◦ **Use Herbs for Flavor**: Enhance your dishes with herbs like mint and basil instead of relying on citrus for flavor.

4. **Instead of Coffee**:

- **Drink Herbal Teas**: Herbal teas can be soothing and provide various health benefits without the acidity of coffee.
- **Try Chicory Root Coffee**: This coffee substitute is caffeine-free and much less acidic.

Sample Meal Plan Avoiding Acidic Foods
Day 1:

- **Breakfast:**
  - Smoothie with spinach, cucumber, apple, and chia seeds
  - A handful of almonds
- **Lunch:**
  - Grilled chicken salad with mixed greens, cucumbers, bell peppers, and a lemon-tahini dressing
  - A serving of quinoa
- **Snack:**
  - Sliced apple with almond butter
- **Dinner:**
  - Baked salmon with a side of steamed broccoli and roasted sweet potatoes
  - A serving of sautéed zucchini and onions

Day 2:

- **Breakfast:**
  - Greek yogurt (plain, unsweetened) with a sprinkle of flaxseeds and a few raspberries
  - Herbal tea (e.g., peppermint tea)
- **Lunch:**
  - Turkey and avocado wrap using a whole grain tortilla, filled with leafy greens and sliced red bell peppers
  - Carrot sticks with hummus
- **Snack:**

- ◦ A small bowl of mixed berries
- • **Dinner:**
  - ◦ Roasted chicken thighs with a side of sautéed kale and garlic
  - ◦ A serving of quinoa with diced onions and parsley

Conclusion

Avoiding acidic foods is crucial for maintaining kidney health, especially for those with weak kidneys. Acidic foods can increase the acid load on the body, leading to conditions like urinary tract infections and kidney stones. By focusing on alkaline foods, lean proteins, and healthy hydration, you can support your kidneys and overall health. Incorporate the strategies and substitutions provided in this chapter to create a balanced, kidney-friendly diet that promotes long-term well-being.

Chapter 8: Avoiding Dairy Products for Kidney Health
Understanding the Impact of Dairy Products on Kidney Health
Dairy products, while rich in essential nutrients such as calcium and protein, can pose significant risks for individuals with compromised kidney function. The consumption of dairy products can exacerbate kidney problems due to their high levels of certain minerals and potential to increase acid load in the body. This chapter will explore why dairy products can be harmful to kidney health and provide alternatives that align with a kidney-friendly diet.

Explanation of Why Dairy Products Are Harmful to Kidney Health

1. **High Phosphorus Content:**
    ◦ **Phosphorus and Kidney Function**: Dairy products contain high levels of phosphorus, which healthy kidneys typically filter out of the blood. However, for individuals with impaired kidney function, excess phosphorus can accumulate in the bloodstream, leading to hyperphosphatemia.
    ◦ **Risks of Hyperphosphatemia**: Elevated phosphorus levels can lead to calcification of blood vessels, joints, and tissues, increasing the risk of cardiovascular diseases and weakening bones by pulling calcium out of them.
2. **High Calcium Content:**
    ◦ **Calcium Overload**: While calcium is necessary for bone health, excessive intake can be problematic for those with kidney disease. Damaged kidneys may not be able to excrete excess calcium, leading to hypercalcemia.

- **Risks of Hypercalcemia**: High levels of calcium in the blood can cause muscle weakness, kidney stones, and impaired kidney function.

3. **Protein Load**:
   - **Excessive Protein**: Dairy products are a significant source of protein. While protein is essential, too much can place a strain on the kidneys, especially if they are already compromised. Excess protein intake can accelerate the progression of kidney disease by increasing the workload on the kidneys.
   - **Nitrogenous Waste**: High protein intake results in the production of more nitrogenous waste, which the kidneys must filter. This can lead to an accumulation of waste products in the blood if kidney function is impaired.

4. **Sodium Content**:
   - **Hidden Sodium**: Many dairy products, especially processed ones like cheese and flavored yogurts, contain high levels of sodium. Excessive sodium can lead to high blood pressure and fluid retention, both of which are harmful to kidney health.
   - **Risks of High Sodium Intake**: High sodium intake exacerbates hypertension, increasing the risk of cardiovascular diseases and further damaging the kidneys.

5. **Lactose Intolerance**:
   - **Digestive Issues**: Many individuals are lactose intolerant, meaning they lack the enzyme lactase needed to digest lactose, the sugar found in milk. This can lead to digestive issues such as bloating, gas, and diarrhea.
   - **Secondary Effects**: Digestive discomfort and inflammation caused by lactose intolerance can exacerbate other health issues and stress the kidneys.

Alternatives to Dairy That Align with the Kidney-Friendly Diet

1. **Plant-Based Milks:**
   - **Almond Milk:** Low in phosphorus and potassium, almond milk is a good alternative to cow's milk. It is also low in calories and can be fortified with calcium and vitamin D.
   - **Oat Milk:** Oat milk is naturally low in fat and can be fortified with essential vitamins and minerals. It has a creamy texture, making it suitable for various culinary uses.
   - **Rice Milk:** Rice milk is one of the least allergenic alternatives and is low in potassium and phosphorus. It can be fortified with calcium and vitamin D.
   - **Coconut Milk:** Rich in healthy fats, coconut milk is a versatile dairy alternative. However, it should be consumed in moderation due to its higher fat content.
2. **Plant-Based Yogurts:**
   - **Almond Yogurt:** Made from almond milk, it is low in potassium and phosphorus and can be a good source of probiotics if fortified.
   - **Coconut Yogurt:** Made from coconut milk, it is creamy and rich, providing a good alternative to traditional yogurt. Ensure it is low in added sugars.
   - **Soy Yogurt:** While higher in protein, soy yogurt can be a good alternative if chosen wisely, ensuring it is low in phosphorus and potassium.
3. **Plant-Based Cheeses:**
   - **Nutritional Yeast:** A deactivated yeast, it has a cheesy flavor and is rich in B vitamins. It can be used as a cheese substitute in various dishes.
   - **Cashew Cheese:** Made from blended cashews, it is creamy and can be flavored to mimic traditional cheese.
   - **Soy Cheese:** Available in various flavors and forms, soy cheese can be a good alternative, but it is essential to choose varieties low in sodium and phosphorus.
4. **Other Plant-Based Alternatives:**

- **Tofu**: A versatile ingredient, tofu can be used in place of dairy in many recipes. It is low in fat and can be fortified with calcium.
- **Hemp Milk**: Made from hemp seeds, it is rich in omega-3 and omega-6 fatty acids. It can be fortified with essential nutrients.

5. **Homemade Dairy Alternatives**:
   - **Homemade Almond Milk**: Soak almonds overnight, blend with water, and strain to create fresh almond milk. This ensures there are no added sugars or preservatives.
   - **Homemade Cashew Cream**: Soak cashews, blend with water, and use as a creamy base for sauces and soups.
   - **Homemade Coconut Milk**: Blend shredded coconut with water and strain to create fresh coconut milk.

Practical Examples and Recipes

1. **Breakfast**:
   - **Smoothie Bowl**: Blend almond milk with spinach, banana, and berries. Top with chia seeds and sliced almonds.
   - **Oatmeal**: Cook oats in oat milk and top with fresh fruits and a sprinkle of cinnamon.

2. **Lunch**:
   - **Vegetable Stir-Fry**: Use tofu as a protein source, stir-fried with a mix of colorful vegetables and a splash of soy sauce.
   - **Salad with Cashew Dressing**: A mixed green salad topped with a creamy cashew dressing (blend soaked cashews with lemon juice, garlic, and water).

3. **Snack**:
   - **Coconut Yogurt with Berries**: A serving of coconut yogurt topped with fresh berries and a handful of nuts.
   - **Almond Cheese and Crackers**: Slices of almond cheese served with whole-grain crackers.

4. **Dinner:**
   - **Stuffed Bell Peppers**: Bell peppers stuffed with quinoa, black beans, corn, and topped with nutritional yeast.
   - **Creamy Coconut Curry**: Vegetables and tofu cooked in a creamy coconut milk curry, served with a side of brown rice.

Benefits of Dairy Alternatives

1. **Reduced Phosphorus and Potassium:**
   - **Lower Mineral Load**: Plant-based alternatives typically have lower levels of phosphorus and potassium, reducing the burden on the kidneys.
2. **Improved Digestive Health:**
   - **Easier Digestion**: Dairy alternatives are easier to digest for those who are lactose intolerant, preventing digestive discomfort and inflammation.
3. **Better Nutrient Profile:**
   - **Fortified Options**: Many plant-based alternatives are fortified with essential vitamins and minerals, providing necessary nutrients without the risks associated with dairy.
4. **Lower Sodium:**
   - **Healthier Choices**: Plant-based alternatives often have lower sodium content, helping to manage blood pressure and reduce the risk of fluid retention.
5. **Heart Health:**
   - **Healthy Fats**: Many dairy alternatives, such as those made from nuts and seeds, provide healthy fats that support cardiovascular health.

Conclusion

Avoiding dairy products is a crucial step in maintaining kidney health, especially for those with compromised kidney function. Dairy products can contribute to high phosphorus and calcium levels, increased acid load, and digestive issues. By incorporating plant-based alternatives such as almond milk, coconut yogurt, and cashew cheese, individuals can enjoy the benefits of essential nutrients without the associated risks. Embrace these alternatives to support your kidney health and overall well-being, and explore the variety of delicious and nutritious options available.

Author's Note:

Hello,

Personally, I avoid all dairy whether it is plant based or regular because it contains sugar, but potential pesticides. I never liked dairy, so if you want to get dairy products, please be cautious here too.

-Matthew Petchinsky

Chapter 9: Benefits of Ginger Tea and Herbal Teas

Introduction

Incorporating herbal teas into your diet can offer significant benefits for kidney health and overall well-being. Among these, ginger tea stands out for its exceptional medicinal properties, particularly in reducing inflammation and supporting urinary tract health. This chapter will provide a detailed overview of the benefits of ginger tea, recommend other herbal teas for kidney health, and emphasize the importance of avoiding sodas and sugary drinks.

Detailed Overview of Ginger Tea's Benefits

1. **Anti-Inflammatory Properties**:
   - **Reducing Inflammation**: Ginger contains potent anti-inflammatory compounds called gingerols and shogaols. These compounds inhibit the production of pro-inflammatory cytokines and enzymes, helping to reduce inflammation in the body.
   - **Kidney Health**: Chronic inflammation is a significant contributor to the progression of kidney disease. By reducing inflammation, ginger tea can help protect the kidneys from further damage and improve their function.

2. **Antioxidant Effects**:
   - **Neutralizing Free Radicals**: Ginger is rich in antioxidants, which help neutralize free radicals and prevent oxidative stress. Oxidative stress can damage kidney cells and contribute to the development of kidney disease.
   - **Supporting Overall Health**: The antioxidants in ginger tea support overall health by protecting cells from damage and reducing the risk of chronic diseases.

3. **Digestive Health**:

- **Aiding Digestion**: Ginger tea stimulates the production of digestive enzymes and increases bile production, aiding in the digestion of food and the absorption of nutrients.
- **Reducing Nausea**: Ginger is well-known for its ability to reduce nausea and vomiting, making it beneficial for individuals undergoing treatments that affect the digestive system.

4. **Urinary Tract Health**:
   - **Antimicrobial Properties**: Ginger has natural antimicrobial properties that help prevent and fight infections. Regular consumption of ginger tea can help reduce the risk of urinary tract infections (UTIs).
   - **Diuretic Effect**: Ginger tea has a mild diuretic effect, promoting urine production and helping flush out toxins and bacteria from the urinary tract, which can prevent the formation of kidney stones and UTIs.

5. **Pain Relief**:
   - **Alleviating Pain**: The anti-inflammatory properties of ginger can help alleviate pain associated with inflammatory conditions, including arthritis and muscle pain. This can indirectly benefit kidney health by reducing the need for pain medications, which can have adverse effects on the kidneys.

6. **Blood Sugar Regulation**:
   - **Stabilizing Blood Sugar**: Ginger has been shown to improve insulin sensitivity and help regulate blood sugar levels. Maintaining stable blood sugar levels is crucial for preventing diabetes, a leading cause of kidney disease.

Other Recommended Herbal Teas for Kidney Health

1. **Dandelion Root Tea**:

- **Detoxifying the Kidneys**: Dandelion root tea acts as a natural diuretic, promoting urine production and helping flush out toxins from the kidneys.
- **Rich in Nutrients**: It contains vitamins A, C, and K, as well as minerals like iron, potassium, and calcium, which support overall kidney function.

2. **Nettle Leaf Tea:**
   - **Reducing Inflammation**: Nettle leaf tea has anti-inflammatory properties that can help reduce inflammation in the kidneys and urinary tract.
   - **Supporting Detoxification**: It promotes the elimination of waste products from the body and supports kidney health.

3. **Horsetail Tea:**
   - **Diuretic Properties**: Horsetail tea is a natural diuretic that increases urine output and helps flush out excess fluids and toxins.
   - **Silica Content**: It is rich in silica, which supports the health of connective tissues, including those in the kidneys.

4. **Parsley Tea:**
   - **Natural Diuretic**: Parsley tea increases urine production and helps cleanse the kidneys by flushing out toxins and reducing the risk of kidney stones.
   - **Rich in Antioxidants**: It contains antioxidants that protect kidney cells from damage.

5. **Marshmallow Root Tea:**
   - **Soothing the Urinary Tract**: Marshmallow root tea has soothing and anti-inflammatory properties that can help alleviate irritation in the urinary tract.
   - **Supporting Kidney Health**: It promotes overall kidney health by reducing inflammation and supporting the body's natural detoxification processes.

6. **Corn Silk Tea:**

- **Reducing Urinary Discomfort**: Corn silk tea is known for its soothing effects on the urinary tract and can help reduce discomfort associated with UTIs.
- **Promoting Diuresis**: It acts as a mild diuretic, increasing urine flow and helping cleanse the kidneys.

Strict Avoidance of Sodas and Sugary Drinks

1. **High Sugar Content**:
   - **Increased Risk of Diabetes**: Sodas and sugary drinks are high in added sugars, which can lead to insulin resistance and the development of type 2 diabetes, a major risk factor for kidney disease.
   - **Weight Gain**: Excessive sugar intake contributes to obesity, which increases the risk of hypertension, diabetes, and subsequent kidney damage.
2. **Phosphoric Acid**:
   - **Phosphorus Overload**: Many sodas, especially colas, contain phosphoric acid, which can lead to an excess of phosphorus in the body. This can result in hyperphosphatemia, causing calcium to be pulled from bones and deposited in blood vessels, joints, and organs, including the kidneys.
   - **Kidney Stones**: Phosphoric acid can also contribute to the formation of kidney stones.
3. **Artificial Additives**:
   - **Chemical Additives**: Sodas and sugary drinks often contain artificial colors, flavors, and preservatives, which can be harmful to kidney health. These chemicals can increase the toxic load on the kidneys, making it harder for them to function properly.
   - **Caffeine**: Many sodas contain caffeine, which can act as a diuretic, leading to dehydration and putting additional strain on the kidneys.

4. **Acid Load:**
    - **Increased Acidity**: Sodas are highly acidic, which can increase the body's acid load and burden the kidneys. Over time, this can lead to metabolic acidosis, a condition where the body produces too much acid or when the kidneys are not removing enough acid from the body.

Practical Tips for Incorporating Herbal Teas into Your Diet

1. **Daily Routine:**
    - **Morning Boost**: Start your day with a cup of ginger tea to kickstart your metabolism and reduce inflammation.
    - **Midday Refreshment**: Enjoy a cup of dandelion root tea or nettle leaf tea in the afternoon to support kidney detoxification and overall health.
2. **Flavor Enhancements:**
    - **Natural Sweeteners**: Use a small amount of honey or stevia to sweeten your herbal teas if needed, avoiding refined sugars.
    - **Citrus Zest**: Add a slice of lemon or orange zest to your tea for a refreshing twist without increasing acidity.
3. **Hydration Balance:**
    - **Alternating Teas**: Alternate between different herbal teas throughout the day to enjoy a variety of health benefits.
    - **Adequate Water Intake**: Ensure you're also drinking plenty of water alongside herbal teas to maintain proper hydration.
4. **Herbal Tea Recipes:**
    - **Ginger and Turmeric Tea**: Combine fresh ginger slices with a pinch of turmeric powder, steep in hot water, and add a dash of honey for a powerful anti-inflammatory drink.

- ○ **Nettle and Mint Tea**: Mix dried nettle leaves with fresh mint leaves, steep in hot water, and enjoy a refreshing and detoxifying beverage.

Conclusion

Incorporating ginger tea and other herbal teas into your diet can provide substantial benefits for kidney health. Ginger tea, with its anti-inflammatory, antioxidant, and digestive health properties, stands out as a particularly beneficial option. Other herbal teas, such as dandelion root, nettle leaf, and parsley tea, also support kidney function and over-all health. By strictly avoiding sodas and sugary drinks, you can reduce the risk of diabetes, obesity, and kidney damage, further protecting your kidneys. Embrace the natural healing properties of herbal teas to support your kidney health and enhance your overall well-being.

Author's Note:

Hello,

Herbal Teas are an amazing option, you can even get an Herbal Tea called Tazo Vanilla Caramel Chai tea which is one of my favorites. I recommend it, you can test every tea under the sun, it is all about your taste, as long as you do not add sweeteners to it.

All teas you drink have to be "Bland" as we are calling it because of the lack of sweeteners that we are all used to. You will not like it at first but if you keep on a consistence basis(everyday), you will get used to the tastes without the sweeteners.

I recommend when it comes to ginger tea, warm is up for two minutes if you want it warm in the winter, and cold in the summer to keep your body in a cool balance.

-Matthew Petchinsky

Chapter 10: Prevention of Kidney Stones

Understanding Kidney Stones

Kidney stones are hard deposits made of minerals and salts that form inside the kidneys. They can cause severe pain and discomfort and may lead to serious health complications if not managed properly. The formation of kidney stones is influenced by dietary factors, hydration levels, and genetic predisposition. Adopting a kidney-friendly diet is a crucial step in preventing the formation of kidney stones and maintaining overall kidney health.

How the Kidney-Friendly Diet Helps Prevent the Formation of Kidney Stones

1. **Proper Hydration:**
   - **Increased Water Intake:** Staying well-hydrated dilutes the substances in urine that lead to stones. Drinking plenty of fluids, especially water, helps flush out minerals and toxins before they can form stones.
   - **Alkaline Water:** Consuming alkaline water helps maintain the body's pH balance and reduces the acidity of urine, lowering the risk of stone formation.
2. **Reducing Oxalate-Rich Foods:**
   - **Oxalate and Stones:** Oxalates are naturally occurring substances in certain foods. When combined with calcium in urine, they can form calcium oxalate stones. A kidney-friendly diet involves moderating the intake of high-oxalate foods.
   - **Balancing Calcium and Oxalates:** Ensuring an adequate but not excessive intake of calcium helps bind oxalates in the gut rather than in the kidneys, reducing stone formation.

3. **Limiting Sodium Intake:**
    ◦ **Sodium and Calcium**: High sodium intake increases calcium levels in the urine, which can lead to stone formation. A low-sodium diet helps maintain normal calcium levels in the urine and reduces the risk of stones.
4. **Moderate Protein Consumption:**
    ◦ **Protein and Acid Production**: Excessive consumption of animal protein can increase uric acid levels and reduce citrate levels, promoting the formation of uric acid and calcium stones. Moderating protein intake helps prevent this.
5. **Increasing Citrate-Rich Foods:**
    ◦ **Citrate and Stones**: Citrate is a natural inhibitor of stone formation. Consuming foods high in citrate, such as lemons and limes, helps prevent stone formation by binding with calcium in the urine.
6. **Avoiding Sugar and Sweetened Beverages:**
    ◦ **Sugar and Stones**: High sugar intake can increase the risk of kidney stones by causing an imbalance in calcium and phosphate levels. Avoiding sugary drinks and foods helps reduce this risk.

Specific Dietary Recommendations to Avoid Stone-Forming Foods

1. **Hydration:**
    ◦ **Daily Water Intake**: Aim to drink at least 2-3 liters of water per day. Spread your water intake throughout the day to maintain consistent hydration levels.
    ◦ **Herbal Teas**: Include herbal teas like ginger tea and dandelion tea, which support kidney health and hydration.
2. **Foods to Limit or Avoid:**
    ◦ **High-Oxalate Foods:**
        ▪ Spinach

- Rhubarb
- Beets
- Nuts (especially almonds and peanuts)
- Chocolate
- Sweet potatoes
  - High-Sodium Foods:
    - Processed meats (bacon, sausage)
    - Packaged snacks (chips, pretzels)
    - Canned soups and vegetables
    - Fast food and restaurant meals
  - High-Sugar Foods and Beverages:
    - Sodas
    - Fruit juices with added sugars
    - Candies and desserts
  - High-Purine Foods (for uric acid stones):
    - Red meat
    - Organ meats
    - Shellfish
    - Certain fish (sardines, anchovies)

3. Foods to Include:
   - Citrate-Rich Foods:
     - **Citrus Fruits:** Lemons, limes, oranges, and grapefruits are high in citrate and help prevent stone formation.
     - **Berries:** Strawberries, blueberries, and raspberries.
   - Calcium-Rich Foods:
     - **Low-Oxalate Leafy Greens:** Kale, broccoli.
     - **Calcium-Fortified Foods:** Fortified plant-based milks (almond, soy, rice).
   - Low-Oxalate Vegetables:
     - Bell Peppers
     - Zucchini
     - Cauliflower

- Healthy Fats:
  - Avocados
  - Olive Oil
  - Flaxseeds
- Lean Proteins:
  - **Chicken and Turkey**: Skinless and grilled or baked.
  - **Fish**: Salmon, mackerel, and other fatty fish high in omega-3 fatty acids.
  - **Plant-Based Proteins**: Lentils, chickpeas, and other legumes in moderation.

4. **Meal Planning**:
   - **Balanced Meals**: Ensure each meal includes a mix of lean protein, healthy fats, and a variety of fruits and vegetables.
   - **Portion Control**: Keep portion sizes moderate to avoid excessive intake of any particular nutrient that might contribute to stone formation.
   - **Regular Meals**: Eat at regular intervals to help regulate metabolism and prevent excessive consumption of stone-forming foods.

5. **Cooking Methods**:
   - **Healthy Preparation**: Grill, bake, steam, or sauté foods instead of frying. Use minimal oil and salt.
   - **Flavor with Herbs**: Use herbs and spices for flavor instead of high-sodium condiments.

Sample Meal Plan for Preventing Kidney Stones
Day 1:

- **Breakfast:**
  - Smoothie with kale, cucumber, lemon, and chia seeds
  - A handful of almonds
- **Lunch:**

- ◦ Grilled chicken breast with a side salad (mixed greens, bell peppers, cucumbers) dressed with olive oil and lemon juice
  - ◦ A serving of quinoa
- **Snack:**
  - ◦ Sliced apple with almond butter
- **Dinner:**
  - ◦ Baked salmon with a side of steamed broccoli and sweet potatoes
  - ◦ A serving of sautéed zucchini with garlic

Day 2:

- **Breakfast:**
  - ◦ Greek yogurt (plain, unsweetened) with a sprinkle of flax-seeds and a few raspberries
  - ◦ Herbal tea (e.g., peppermint tea)
- **Lunch:**
  - ◦ Turkey and avocado wrap using a whole grain tortilla, filled with leafy greens and sliced red bell peppers
  - ◦ Carrot sticks with hummus
- **Snack:**
  - ◦ A small bowl of mixed berries
- **Dinner:**
  - ◦ Roasted chicken thighs with a side of sautéed kale and garlic
  - ◦ A serving of quinoa with diced onions and parsley

Conclusion

Preventing kidney stones is an integral part of maintaining kidney health. A kidney-friendly diet that emphasizes proper hydration, balanced nutrient intake, and the avoidance of stone-forming foods can significantly reduce the risk of developing kidney stones. By incorporating the dietary recommendations and meal plans outlined in this chapter, you can take proactive steps to support your kidney health and prevent the formation of kidney stones. Embrace these guidelines to enjoy a healthy, balanced diet that promotes long-term well-being and optimal kidney function.

Author's Note:

If your kidney is severely damaged like mine, you must remove any acidic fruits, as well as those full of potassium. Be careful please.

-Matthew Petchinsky

Chapter 11: Urinary Tract Infection (UTI) Prevention
Understanding Urinary Tract Infections (UTIs)

Urinary tract infections (UTIs) are common infections that affect the urinary system, including the bladder, urethra, ureters, and kidneys. They are typically caused by bacteria, such as Escherichia coli (E. coli), entering the urinary tract. UTIs can cause symptoms such as frequent urination, pain or burning during urination, and lower abdominal pain. If left untreated, they can lead to serious complications, including kidney infections. Preventing UTIs involves maintaining proper hygiene, staying hydrated, and adopting a diet that supports urinary tract health.

Role of the Diet in Reducing the Risk of UTIs

1. **Maintaining Urinary pH Balance:**
   - **Alkaline Diet**: Consuming an alkaline diet helps maintain the pH balance of the urine, making it less acidic. This creates an environment that is less conducive to bacterial growth, thereby reducing the risk of UTIs.

2. **Hydration:**
   - **Increased Fluid Intake**: Staying well-hydrated helps flush out bacteria from the urinary tract, reducing the likelihood of infection. Drinking plenty of water ensures that the urinary tract is regularly cleansed, preventing the accumulation of bacteria.
   - **Frequent Urination**: Proper hydration encourages frequent urination, which helps expel bacteria from the bladder before they can cause an infection.

3. **Nutrient-Rich Foods:**
   - **Vitamins and Minerals**: Certain vitamins and minerals, such as vitamin C and zinc, support the immune system and help the body fight off infections, including UTIs.

Consuming a diet rich in these nutrients strengthens the body's defenses against bacterial invasion.

4. **Probiotic-Rich Foods:**
   - **Gut Health**: Probiotics promote a healthy balance of bacteria in the gut, which can influence the bacterial balance in the urinary tract. A healthy gut microbiome helps prevent the overgrowth of harmful bacteria that can cause UTIs.

Foods and Drinks That Support Urinary Tract Health

1. **Cranberries:**
   - **Cranberry Juice**: Cranberries contain compounds called proanthocyanidins that prevent bacteria from adhering to the walls of the urinary tract. Drinking unsweetened cranberry juice or taking cranberry supplements can help reduce the risk of UTIs.

2. **Blueberries:**
   - **Antioxidant-Rich**: Blueberries, like cranberries, contain antioxidants and compounds that prevent bacteria from adhering to the urinary tract lining. Consuming fresh blueberries or adding them to smoothies can support urinary tract health.

3. **Probiotics:**
   - **Yogurt**: Consuming plain, unsweetened yogurt with live active cultures provides beneficial bacteria that support a healthy urinary tract.
   - **Kefir**: Kefir is a fermented milk drink that is rich in probiotics. It can be a beneficial addition to your diet to promote urinary tract health.

4. **High-Fiber Foods:**
   - **Whole Grains**: Foods like oats, quinoa, and brown rice are high in fiber, which supports digestive health and helps prevent constipation. Constipation can contribute to the

development of UTIs by putting pressure on the urinary tract and hindering the complete emptying of the bladder.

◦ **Fruits and Vegetables**: Eating a variety of fruits and vegetables, such as apples, pears, carrots, and leafy greens, ensures adequate fiber intake and supports overall digestive health.

5. **Water-Rich Foods**:

◦ **Cucumbers**: Cucumbers have a high water content, which helps keep the body hydrated and supports the regular flushing of the urinary tract.

◦ **Watermelon**: Watermelon is another hydrating fruit that can help cleanse the urinary system and prevent infections.

6. **Herbal Teas**:

◦ **Dandelion Tea**: Dandelion tea acts as a natural diuretic, promoting urine production and helping flush out bacteria from the urinary tract.

◦ **Nettle Tea**: Nettle tea has anti-inflammatory properties and supports urinary tract health by promoting regular urination.

◦ **Ginger Tea**: Ginger tea has antimicrobial and anti-inflammatory properties that can help prevent and manage UTIs.

7. **Citrus Fruits**:

◦ **Lemons and Limes**: Citrus fruits like lemons and limes are rich in vitamin C, which boosts the immune system and increases the acidity of the urine, creating an environment that is less favorable for bacterial growth.

Practical Tips for Incorporating UTI-Preventive Foods and Drinks into Your Diet

1. **Hydration Routine**:

- **Morning Hydration**: Start your day with a glass of warm water with a splash of lemon juice to kickstart your metabolism and hydrate your body.
- **Consistent Fluid Intake**: Carry a water bottle with you throughout the day to ensure you're drinking enough water. Aim for at least 2-3 liters of water daily.

2. **Balanced Meals:**
   - **Include Probiotics**: Add a serving of plain yogurt or kefir to your breakfast or as a snack to ensure you're getting beneficial bacteria.
   - **High-Fiber Diet**: Incorporate whole grains, fruits, and vegetables into each meal to support digestive health and prevent constipation.

3. **Snack Smart:**
   - **Cranberry and Blueberry Snacks**: Keep dried cranberries (without added sugar) and fresh blueberries on hand for a quick, nutritious snack.
   - **Hydrating Snacks**: Snack on cucumber slices or watermelon chunks to stay hydrated and support urinary tract health.

4. **Herbal Teas:**
   - **Daily Herbal Tea**: Make a habit of drinking a cup of herbal tea, such as dandelion or nettle tea, in the afternoon or evening to promote urinary tract health.
   - **Tea Blends**: Experiment with different blends of herbal teas to find flavors you enjoy while reaping the health benefits.

5. **Citrus Boost:**
   - **Add Citrus to Water**: Add slices of lemon or lime to your water for a refreshing and vitamin C-rich drink.
   - **Citrus in Meals**: Use lemon or lime juice as a dressing for salads or to flavor fish and other dishes.

Sample Meal Plan for UTI Prevention

Day 1:

- **Breakfast:**
  - Greek yogurt (plain, unsweetened) topped with fresh blueberries and a sprinkle of chia seeds
  - A glass of water with a splash of lemon juice
- **Lunch:**
  - Grilled chicken salad with mixed greens, cucumbers, carrots, and a lemon-tahini dressing
  - A serving of quinoa
- **Snack:**
  - A handful of dried cranberries (without added sugar)
- **Dinner:**
  - Baked salmon with a side of steamed broccoli and sweet potatoes
  - A serving of brown rice
- **Evening:**
  - A cup of nettle tea

Day 2:

- **Breakfast:**
  - Smoothie with spinach, cucumber, apple, and chia seeds
  - A glass of water with a splash of lime juice
- **Lunch:**
  - Turkey and avocado wrap using a whole grain tortilla, filled with leafy greens and sliced bell peppers
  - Carrot sticks with hummus
- **Snack:**
  - Sliced apple with almond butter
- **Dinner:**
  - Roasted chicken thighs with a side of sautéed kale and garlic

- ◦ A serving of quinoa with diced onions and parsley
  - **Evening:**
    - ◦ A cup of dandelion tea

Conclusion

Preventing urinary tract infections is vital for maintaining overall kidney health. A diet rich in hydrating fluids, high-fiber foods, probiotics, and specific fruits and vegetables can significantly reduce the risk of UTIs. Incorporating foods and drinks that support urinary tract health, such as cranberries, blueberries, probiotics, and herbal teas, into your daily routine can help maintain a healthy urinary system. By following the dietary recommendations and tips provided in this chapter, you can take proactive steps to prevent UTIs and support long-term urinary tract health.

Chapter 12: Preventing Kidney Infections

Understanding Kidney Infections

Kidney infections, also known as pyelonephritis, occur when bacteria travel from the bladder up to the kidneys. This can lead to severe complications if not managed properly. Maintaining a healthy diet and lifestyle is crucial in preventing kidney infections and supporting overall kidney health. This chapter will explore how an alkaline diet and proper hydration can prevent kidney infections and recommend additional lifestyle changes to enhance kidney health.

How an Alkaline Diet and Proper Hydration Can Prevent Kidney Infections

1. **Alkaline Diet:**
   - **Balancing pH Levels:** An alkaline diet helps maintain a balanced pH in the body, reducing the acidity of the urine. This creates an environment that is less conducive to bacterial growth, thereby reducing the risk of infections.
   - **Anti-Inflammatory Properties:** Alkaline foods, such as leafy greens, vegetables, and certain fruits, have anti-inflammatory properties that help reduce inflammation in the kidneys and urinary tract, lowering the risk of infection.
   - **Nutrient-Rich Foods:** Alkaline foods are rich in essential vitamins and minerals that support immune function and overall health. For instance, leafy greens like spinach and kale are high in vitamins A and C, which boost the immune system.

2. **Proper Hydration:**
   - **Flushing Out Bacteria:** Drinking plenty of fluids, especially water, helps flush out bacteria from the urinary tract,

reducing the risk of infection. Proper hydration ensures that the kidneys can efficiently filter and excrete waste products and bacteria.

- **Diluting Urine**: Adequate water intake dilutes the urine, making it less likely for bacteria to thrive. This dilution also helps prevent the formation of kidney stones, which can create an environment for bacterial growth.
- **Alkaline Water**: Drinking alkaline water can help neutralize body acidity and support kidney function. Alkaline water provides essential electrolytes that help maintain hydration and pH balance.

Alkaline Foods to Include in Your Diet

1. **Vegetables**:
   - **Leafy Greens**: Spinach, kale, Swiss chard, and collard greens.
   - **Cruciferous Vegetables**: Broccoli, cauliflower, Brussels sprouts, and cabbage.
   - **Root Vegetables**: Carrots, beets, sweet potatoes, and radishes.
   - **Other Vegetables**: Cucumbers, zucchini, bell peppers, and celery.
2. **Fruits** (in moderation due to natural sugars):
   - **Berries**: Strawberries, blueberries, raspberries, and blackberries.
   - **Citrus Fruits**: Lemons, limes, and grapefruits.
   - **Other Fruits**: Apples, pears, peaches, and cherries.
3. **Nuts and Seeds**:
   - **Almonds**
   - **Chia Seeds**
   - **Flaxseeds**
   - **Pumpkin Seeds**

4. **Legumes** (in moderation):
     - Lentils
     - Chickpeas
     - Black Beans
     - Kidney Beans
5. **Herbs and Spices:**
     - Basil
     - Parsley
     - Cilantro
     - Garlic
     - Ginger
6. **Healthy Fats:**
     - Avocados
     - Olive Oil
     - Coconut Oil
7. **Whole Grains:**
     - Quinoa
     - Buckwheat
     - Millet

Additional Lifestyle Changes to Support Kidney Health

1. **Maintaining Proper Hygiene:**
     - **Personal Hygiene:** Practice good personal hygiene, such as wiping front to back after using the bathroom, to prevent bacteria from entering the urinary tract.
     - **Shower Instead of Bathing:** Taking showers instead of baths can reduce the risk of bacterial contamination.
2. **Regular Physical Activity:**
     - **Exercise:** Regular exercise helps maintain a healthy weight, reduces blood pressure, and improves circulation, all of which support kidney health.

- ◦ **Avoid Prolonged Sitting**: Avoid sitting for prolonged periods as it can reduce blood flow to the kidneys.

3. **Healthy Eating Habits**:
    - ◦ **Balanced Diet**: Follow a balanced diet rich in fruits, vegetables, lean proteins, and whole grains to support overall health.
    - ◦ **Limit Processed Foods**: Avoid processed foods high in sodium, sugars, and unhealthy fats that can strain the kidneys.

4. **Avoiding Harmful Substances**:
    - ◦ **Tobacco and Alcohol**: Avoid smoking and limit alcohol consumption, as these substances can damage the kidneys and reduce their ability to filter waste.
    - ◦ **Medications**: Use medications responsibly, and avoid over-the-counter pain relievers like NSAIDs (ibuprofen, naproxen) unless prescribed by a healthcare provider, as they can harm the kidneys.

5. **Managing Chronic Conditions**:
    - ◦ **Blood Pressure and Diabetes**: Keep chronic conditions such as high blood pressure and diabetes under control, as these are leading causes of kidney disease.
    - ◦ **Regular Check-Ups**: Regular medical check-ups help monitor kidney function and manage underlying health issues.

6. **Stress Management**:
    - ◦ **Relaxation Techniques**: Practice relaxation techniques such as yoga, meditation, and deep breathing exercises to reduce stress, which can negatively impact kidney function.
    - ◦ **Adequate Sleep**: Ensure you get enough sleep, as proper rest is crucial for overall health and kidney function.

7. **Dietary Supplements**:

- **Probiotics**: Consider taking probiotics to support gut health and the immune system, which can help prevent infections.
- **Vitamins and Minerals**: Ensure adequate intake of essential vitamins and minerals through diet or supplements, as advised by a healthcare provider.

Practical Tips for Incorporating Alkaline Foods and Proper Hydration

1. **Daily Routine**:
   - **Morning Hydration**: Start your day with a glass of warm water with a splash of lemon juice to kickstart your metabolism and hydrate your body.
   - **Consistent Fluid Intake**: Drink water throughout the day to maintain hydration levels. Carry a water bottle with you to ensure you are drinking enough.
2. **Meal Planning**:
   - **Balanced Meals**: Plan meals that include a variety of alkaline vegetables, lean proteins, and healthy fats. Incorporate fruits in moderation to avoid excessive sugar intake.
   - **Portion Control**: Keep portion sizes moderate to avoid overeating and ensure a balanced intake of nutrients.
3. **Cooking Methods**:
   - **Healthy Preparation**: Use grilling, baking, steaming, and sautéing as primary cooking methods to retain nutrients and minimize added fats.
   - **Flavor with Herbs**: Enhance the flavor of your meals with herbs and spices instead of high-sodium condiments.
4. **Snacking**:
   - **Healthy Snacks**: Choose healthy snacks such as raw vegetables, nuts, seeds, and fruits. Avoid processed snacks high in sodium and sugar.

5. **Herbal Teas:**
    - **Incorporate Herbal Teas:** Drink herbal teas like ginger tea, dandelion tea, and nettle tea, which support kidney health and provide hydration.

Sample Meal Plan for Preventing Kidney Infections
Day 1:

- **Breakfast:**
    - Smoothie with spinach, cucumber, lemon, and chia seeds
    - A handful of almonds
- **Lunch:**
    - Grilled chicken breast with a side salad (mixed greens, bell peppers, cucumbers) dressed with olive oil and lemon juice
    - A serving of quinoa
- **Snack:**
    - Sliced apple with almond butter
- **Dinner:**
    - Baked salmon with a side of steamed broccoli and sweet potatoes
    - A serving of sautéed zucchini with garlic

Day 2:

- **Breakfast:**
    - Greek yogurt (plain, unsweetened) with a sprinkle of flax-seeds and a few raspberries
    - Herbal tea (e.g., peppermint tea)
- **Lunch:**
    - Turkey and avocado wrap using a whole grain tortilla, filled with leafy greens and sliced red bell peppers
    - Carrot sticks with hummus
- **Snack:**

- A small bowl of mixed berries
- **Dinner:**
    - Roasted chicken thighs with a side of sautéed kale and garlic
    - A serving of quinoa with diced onions and parsley

Conclusion

Preventing kidney infections is essential for maintaining overall kidney health. An alkaline diet and proper hydration play a significant role in reducing the risk of infections by maintaining a balanced pH, reducing inflammation, and supporting immune function. By incorporating additional lifestyle changes such as proper hygiene, regular physical activity, healthy eating habits, and managing chronic conditions, you can further support your kidney health and prevent infections. Embrace these guidelines to create a balanced, kidney-friendly lifestyle that promotes long-term well-being and optimal kidney function.

Chapter 13: The Science Behind Alkaline Water and Reverse Osmosis

Understanding Alkaline Water

Alkaline water has a higher pH level than regular drinking water, typically around 8 or 9, compared to the neutral pH of 7. The alkaline water's increased pH is achieved by adding minerals such as calcium, potassium, and magnesium, which can have various health benefits, particularly for kidney health.

The Science Supporting Alkaline Water

1. **pH Balance and Acid-Base Homeostasis:**
   - **Acid-Base Homeostasis:** The body maintains a tightly regulated pH balance, crucial for normal cellular function and metabolic processes. The kidneys play a vital role in maintaining this balance by excreting hydrogen ions and reabsorbing bicarbonate from urine.
   - **Alkaline Water's Role:** Drinking alkaline water can help neutralize excess acidity in the body, reducing the burden on the kidneys and promoting overall pH balance. This can be particularly beneficial for individuals with chronic kidney disease (CKD), where the kidneys' ability to maintain acid-base balance is compromised.

2. **Antioxidant Properties:**
   - **Reduction of Oxidative Stress:** Alkaline water has antioxidant properties due to its negative oxidation-reduction potential (ORP). This means it can donate electrons and neutralize reactive oxygen species (ROS), reducing oxidative stress.

- **Kidney Health**: Oxidative stress is a significant contributor to kidney damage and progression of kidney disease. By reducing oxidative stress, alkaline water may help protect kidney cells and improve overall kidney function.

3. **Hydration and Electrolyte Balance:**
   - **Enhanced Hydration**: Alkaline water is believed to be more easily absorbed by the body, leading to better hydration. Proper hydration is crucial for kidney health as it aids in the filtration and excretion of waste products.
   - **Electrolyte Supply**: The minerals in alkaline water, such as calcium, potassium, and magnesium, are essential electrolytes that support various bodily functions, including muscle function, nerve transmission, and fluid balance. These minerals also play a role in maintaining kidney function.

Research Findings on Alkaline Water and Kidney Health

1. **Study on Metabolic Acidosis:**
   - **Background**: Metabolic acidosis is a condition where there is too much acid in the body fluids, often seen in CKD patients. It can lead to muscle wasting, bone disease, and progression of kidney disease.
   - **Findings**: A study published in the Journal of the American Society of Nephrology found that alkali supplementation (including alkaline water) improved metabolic acidosis in CKD patients, leading to better muscle function and slower progression of kidney disease.

2. **Antioxidant Effects Study:**
   - **Background**: Chronic oxidative stress contributes to the development and progression of kidney disease.
   - **Findings**: Research published in Evidence-Based Complementary and Alternative Medicine demonstrated that alkaline water reduced oxidative stress markers in animal

models, suggesting potential protective effects on kidney function.

3. **Hydration and Kidney Function**:
   - **Background**: Proper hydration is essential for maintaining kidney function and preventing kidney stones.
   - **Findings**: Studies have shown that drinking alkaline water improves hydration status and urine output, which can help in the prevention of kidney stones and support overall kidney health.

Understanding Reverse Osmosis Water

Reverse osmosis (RO) is a water purification process that uses a semi-permeable membrane to remove ions, molecules, and larger particles from drinking water. This process is highly effective in producing clean, pure water by filtering out contaminants that can be harmful to health, including kidney health.

The Science Supporting Reverse Osmosis Water

1. **Removal of Contaminants**:
   - **Heavy Metals and Chemicals**: RO systems effectively remove heavy metals like lead, mercury, and arsenic, as well as chemical contaminants like chlorine, fluoride, and nitrates. These contaminants can cause significant health issues, including kidney damage.
   - **Microorganisms**: RO systems also remove bacteria, viruses, and parasites, reducing the risk of waterborne diseases that can affect kidney health.
2. **Improving Water Quality**:
   - **Reduction of Total Dissolved Solids (TDS)**: RO filtration reduces the level of total dissolved solids in water, which includes organic and inorganic substances that can burden the kidneys.

- ○ **Taste and Odor**: By removing impurities, RO water has an improved taste and odor, encouraging higher water intake, which is essential for kidney health.

3. **Safe for Sensitive Populations**:
   - ○ **Kidney Patients**: Individuals with compromised kidney function are more susceptible to the adverse effects of water contaminants. RO water provides an added layer of safety by ensuring the water they consume is free from harmful substances.

Research Findings on Reverse Osmosis Water and Kidney Health

1. **Study on Contaminant Removal**:
   - ○ **Background**: Contaminated water can lead to various health issues, including kidney disease.
   - ○ **Findings**: A study published in the Journal of Environmental Science and Health showed that RO systems effectively removed contaminants, significantly improving water quality and reducing health risks associated with contaminated water.

2. **Hydration and Kidney Stones**:
   - ○ **Background**: Proper hydration is critical in preventing kidney stones.
   - ○ **Findings**: Research in the American Journal of Kidney Diseases highlighted that consuming purified water from RO systems improved hydration and reduced the incidence of kidney stones in individuals prone to stone formation.

3. **Long-Term Health Benefits**:
   - ○ **Background**: Long-term exposure to water contaminants can lead to chronic health conditions, including kidney disease.
   - ○ **Findings**: A review in the International Journal of Environmental Research and Public Health concluded that

long-term consumption of RO water is associated with reduced exposure to harmful contaminants, promoting better kidney health and overall well-being.

Combining Alkaline and Reverse Osmosis Water for Optimal Kidney Health

1. **Enhanced Purification and Alkalinity:**
   - **Combination Benefits**: Using an RO system to purify water and then adding minerals to create alkaline water combines the benefits of contaminant removal with the advantages of an alkaline pH. This approach ensures the water is both clean and supportive of kidney health.
2. **Daily Routine:**
   - **Morning Routine**: Start the day with a glass of alkaline water to kickstart hydration and support pH balance.
   - **Throughout the Day**: Alternate between RO water and alkaline water to maintain consistent hydration and electrolyte balance.
3. **Cooking and Food Preparation:**
   - **Using RO Water**: Use RO water for cooking to ensure food is free from contaminants.
   - **Adding Alkaline Water**: Incorporate alkaline water in recipes where appropriate, such as in smoothies or soups, to enhance nutrient absorption and support kidney health.

Practical Tips for Implementing Alkaline and Reverse Osmosis Water

1. **Choosing the Right System:**
   - **RO Systems**: Invest in a high-quality RO system with multi-stage filtration to ensure thorough contaminant removal.

- **Alkaline Water Ionizers**: Consider adding an alkaline water ionizer to your RO system to enhance the pH of the purified water.

2. **Maintenance and Monitoring:**
   - **Regular Maintenance**: Ensure regular maintenance of your RO system to keep it functioning optimally. Replace filters as recommended by the manufacturer.
   - **pH Testing**: Periodically test the pH of your alkaline water to ensure it remains at the desired level.

3. **Hydration Goals:**
   - **Consistent Hydration**: Aim to drink at least 2-3 liters of water daily, using a combination of RO and alkaline water to meet your hydration needs.
   - **Listening to Your Body**: Adjust your water intake based on activity level, climate, and individual health needs.

Conclusion

The science behind alkaline and reverse osmosis water supports their use in promoting kidney health and overall well-being. Alkaline water helps balance pH levels, reduce oxidative stress, and enhance hydration, while reverse osmosis water provides superior purification, removing harmful contaminants. Combining these two types of water offers comprehensive benefits, ensuring that the water you consume is both clean and supportive of optimal kidney function. By understanding the research and implementing these water choices into your daily routine, you can take proactive steps to protect your kidneys and enhance your overall health.

Chapter 14: Benefits of a Meat-Based Diet
Historical Context of Meat-Based Diets and Their Health Benefits

1. **Historical Perspective:**
   - **Ancestral Diets:** Throughout history, humans have consumed meat as a primary food source. Early hunter-gatherer societies relied heavily on meat for its nutrient density and availability. These diets were rich in animal proteins and fats, which provided essential nutrients necessary for survival and development.
   - **Evolutionary Adaptation:** The human digestive system has evolved to efficiently process and utilize nutrients from meat. Our ancestors' reliance on meat contributed to the development of larger brains and smaller guts, as meat is calorie-dense and nutrient-rich, supporting higher energy demands and cognitive function.

2. **Nutritional Value of Meat:**
   - **Complete Protein:** Meat is a complete protein source, containing all essential amino acids required for the body's growth, repair, and maintenance. Amino acids are the building blocks of proteins and are crucial for muscle development, immune function, and enzyme production.
   - **Rich in Micronutrients:** Meat provides essential vitamins and minerals such as B vitamins (B12, niacin, riboflavin), iron, zinc, selenium, and phosphorus. These nutrients play critical roles in various bodily functions, including energy production, immune support, and cellular repair.

3. **Cultural Significance:**
   - **Dietary Staples:** In many cultures, meat has been a staple food, symbolizing wealth, strength, and vitality. Traditional

diets in various regions often emphasize meat as a central component, reflecting its importance in human nutrition.

- **Rituals and Traditions**: Meat consumption has also been integral to many cultural rituals and celebrations, highlighting its significance beyond just sustenance.

How Meat Supports Kidney Health and Overall Wellness

1. **Nutrient Density**:
   - **High-Quality Protein**: Meat provides high-quality protein that is easily absorbed and utilized by the body. Protein is essential for muscle maintenance, tissue repair, and overall bodily functions. Adequate protein intake is particularly important for individuals with kidney issues, as it helps maintain muscle mass and supports recovery.
   - **Iron and Hemoglobin**: Iron from meat (heme iron) is more readily absorbed than non-heme iron from plant sources. Iron is crucial for the production of hemoglobin, which carries oxygen in the blood. Adequate iron levels support energy levels and prevent anemia, a common issue in individuals with kidney disease.
2. **Support for Kidney Health**:
   - **Phosphorus and Potassium Balance**: While it's essential to monitor phosphorus and potassium intake for individuals with kidney disease, lean meats like chicken, turkey, and certain fish can provide necessary nutrients without excessive amounts of these minerals. Proper management of phosphorus and potassium intake can help prevent complications associated with kidney disease.
   - **Anti-Inflammatory Effects**: Omega-3 fatty acids found in fatty fish like salmon and mackerel have anti-inflammatory properties that can reduce inflammation in the kidneys and support overall kidney health.

3. **Overall Wellness:**
  - **Immune Support:** Meat is rich in zinc and selenium, which are vital for immune function. These minerals help the body fight infections and support overall immune health.
  - **Energy and Metabolism:** B vitamins found in meat, such as B12, niacin, and riboflavin, are essential for energy production and metabolic processes. These vitamins support the conversion of food into energy and play a role in maintaining healthy skin, nerves, and digestion.
  - **Muscle Maintenance and Repair:** The protein in meat is crucial for muscle maintenance and repair. Adequate protein intake supports physical activity, recovery from illness, and overall strength.

Specific Benefits of Different Types of Meat

1. **Beef:**
  - **Lean Cuts:** Opt for lean cuts like sirloin, tenderloin, and round steak. These cuts provide high-quality protein with lower fat content.
  - **Iron and B Vitamins:** Beef is an excellent source of heme iron and B vitamins, supporting energy levels and red blood cell production.
2. **Poultry:**
  - **Chicken and Turkey:** Skinless chicken breasts and turkey are low in fat and high in protein. They are also rich in niacin and selenium, supporting immune function and metabolic health.
  - **Versatile and Lean:** Poultry can be prepared in various ways, making it a versatile and healthy addition to the diet.
3. **Fish and Seafood:**

- **Fatty Fish**: Salmon, mackerel, and sardines are rich in omega-3 fatty acids, which have anti-inflammatory properties and support heart and kidney health.
- **Lean Fish**: Cod, haddock, and tilapia are low in fat and high in protein, making them excellent choices for a balanced diet.

4. **Game Meats**:
   - **Venison and Bison**: These meats are lean, high in protein, and rich in essential nutrients like iron and B vitamins. They are also lower in fat compared to conventional meats.
   - **Nutrient-Dense**: Game meats are often considered more nutrient-dense due to their natural diet and active lifestyle.

5. **Organ Meats**:
   - **Liver and Kidneys**: Organ meats are exceptionally rich in vitamins and minerals, including vitamin A, B vitamins, iron, and zinc. However, they should be consumed in moderation due to their high nutrient density.
   - **Digestive Considerations**: Individual tolerance varies, so it's important to monitor how your digestive system responds to organ meats and adjust your intake accordingly.

Incorporating Meat into a Kidney-Friendly Diet

1. **Balanced Meals**:
   - **Portion Control**: Aim for balanced portion sizes to ensure you're getting enough protein without overburdening the kidneys. A typical serving size is about 3-4 ounces of cooked meat.
   - **Complementary Foods**: Pair meat with a variety of vegetables, whole grains, and healthy fats to create well-rounded meals that support overall health and kidney function.

2. **Cooking Methods**:

- ◦ **Healthy Preparation**: Use grilling, baking, roasting, and steaming as primary cooking methods to retain nutrients and minimize added fats.
- ◦ **Avoid Frying**: Frying can add unnecessary fats and create harmful compounds. Opt for healthier cooking methods to maximize the benefits of meat.

3. **Hydration and Supplements**:
- ◦ **Stay Hydrated**: Proper hydration is crucial for kidney health, especially when consuming a higher protein diet. Ensure you drink plenty of water throughout the day.
- ◦ **Consider Supplements**: Depending on your diet and health needs, you might need supplements to ensure you're getting all necessary nutrients. Consult with a healthcare provider to determine if you need additional vitamins or minerals.

Sample Meal Plan Featuring Meat-Based Diet
Day 1:

- **Breakfast:**
  - ◦ Scrambled eggs with spinach and tomatoes
  - ◦ A small serving of smoked salmon
  - ◦ Herbal tea (e.g., ginger tea)
- **Lunch:**
  - ◦ Grilled chicken salad with mixed greens, bell peppers, cucumbers, and a lemon-tahini dressing
  - ◦ A serving of quinoa
- **Snack:**
  - ◦ Greek yogurt (plain, unsweetened) with a handful of almonds
- **Dinner:**
  - ◦ Baked salmon with a side of steamed broccoli and roasted sweet potatoes

  ◦ A serving of brown rice

Day 2:

- **Breakfast:**
  - Omelette with turkey, bell peppers, and onions
  - A small bowl of mixed berries
- **Lunch:**
  - Turkey and avocado wrap using a whole grain tortilla, filled with leafy greens and sliced red bell peppers
  - Carrot sticks with hummus
- **Snack:**
  - A small bowl of mixed nuts
- **Dinner:**
  - Roasted venison with a side of sautéed kale and garlic
  - A serving of wild rice

Conclusion

A meat-based diet, rooted in historical and evolutionary contexts, offers numerous health benefits, particularly for kidney health and overall wellness. Meat provides high-quality protein, essential vitamins, and minerals that support muscle maintenance, immune function, and energy production. By incorporating a variety of meats, including lean cuts of beef, poultry, fish, and game meats, into a balanced diet, you can enjoy these benefits while supporting your kidney health. Use healthy cooking methods, maintain proper hydration, and consider dietary supplements as needed to create a comprehensive, kidney-friendly diet that promotes long-term health and well-being.

Chapter 15: Avoiding Seed Oils
Explanation of Why Seed Oils Are Harmful

Seed oils, also known as vegetable oils, are extracted from seeds and are commonly used in cooking and food processing. These oils include soybean oil, corn oil, sunflower oil, safflower oil, and canola oil. Despite their prevalence in the modern diet, seed oils can have harmful effects on health, particularly for individuals with kidney issues.

1. **High in Omega-6 Fatty Acids**:
    - **Imbalance with Omega-3**: Seed oils are high in omega-6 fatty acids, which, when consumed in excess, can lead to an imbalance with omega-3 fatty acids. This imbalance can promote inflammation, a key factor in the progression of chronic diseases, including kidney disease.
    - **Pro-Inflammatory Effects**: Omega-6 fatty acids can convert into arachidonic acid, which is a precursor to pro-inflammatory molecules. Chronic inflammation can exacerbate kidney damage and contribute to other health issues such as cardiovascular disease and arthritis.

2. **Oxidative Stress**:
    - **Susceptibility to Oxidation**: Seed oils are prone to oxidation due to their high content of polyunsaturated fats. Oxidation produces harmful free radicals that can damage cells and tissues, leading to oxidative stress.
    - **Impact on Kidneys**: Oxidative stress is a significant contributor to kidney damage and the progression of kidney disease. Consuming oxidized fats can increase the burden on the kidneys to filter and excrete these harmful compounds.

3. **Processing and Additives**:
    - **Refining Process**: Many seed oils undergo extensive refining, which involves high heat, chemical solvents, and bleaching agents. This process can strip the oils of beneficial nutrients and introduce harmful compounds.
    - **Additives and Preservatives**: Processed seed oils often contain additives and preservatives that can be detrimental to health, including artificial antioxidants like butylated hydroxytoluene (BHT) and butylated hydroxyanisole (BHA), which are linked to various health risks.
4. **Trans Fats**:
    - **Partial Hydrogenation**: Some seed oils are partially hydrogenated to increase their shelf life and stability, resulting in the formation of trans fats. Trans fats are associated with increased inflammation, insulin resistance, and a higher risk of chronic diseases, including kidney disease.

Alternatives to Seed Oils

1. **Olive Oil**:
    - **Monounsaturated Fats**: Olive oil is rich in monounsaturated fats, which are more stable and less prone to oxidation compared to polyunsaturated fats.
    - **Anti-Inflammatory Properties**: Olive oil contains antioxidants and anti-inflammatory compounds, such as oleocanthal, which can help reduce inflammation and oxidative stress.
    - **Best Use**: Ideal for salad dressings, drizzling over cooked vegetables, and low to medium-heat cooking.
2. **Coconut Oil**:
    - **Saturated Fats**: Coconut oil is composed primarily of saturated fats, making it highly stable and resistant to oxidation.

- **Medium-Chain Triglycerides (MCTs)**: Coconut oil contains medium-chain triglycerides, which are easily metabolized for energy and have been shown to have antimicrobial and metabolic benefits.
- **Best Use**: Suitable for baking, sautéing, and high-heat cooking.

3. **Avocado Oil**:
   - **Monounsaturated Fats**: Similar to olive oil, avocado oil is high in monounsaturated fats, providing stability and health benefits.
   - **Nutrient-Rich**: Avocado oil is rich in vitamins E and K, which support skin health and have antioxidant properties.
   - **Best Use**: Ideal for salad dressings, marinades, and high-heat cooking due to its high smoke point.

4. **Butter and Ghee**:
   - **Natural Saturated Fats**: Butter and ghee (clarified butter) are natural sources of saturated fats that are stable and less likely to oxidize.
   - **Nutrient-Dense**: Butter and ghee contain fat-soluble vitamins such as A, D, E, and K2, which are important for overall health.
   - **Best Use**: Suitable for baking, sautéing, and high-heat cooking.

5. **Animal Fats**:
   - **Tallow and Lard**: Animal fats like beef tallow and pork lard are traditional cooking fats that are high in saturated and monounsaturated fats, making them stable and nutritious.
   - **Natural Source**: These fats are minimally processed and provide essential nutrients.
   - **Best Use**: Ideal for frying, roasting, and baking.

Benefits of Using Healthy Fats for Kidney and Overall Health

1. **Reduced Inflammation**:
   - **Anti-Inflammatory Fats**: Healthy fats, such as those found in olive oil and avocado oil, contain anti-inflammatory properties that can help reduce chronic inflammation. This is particularly beneficial for kidney health, as inflammation plays a key role in the progression of kidney disease.
   - **Balanced Omega Ratios**: By using healthy fats, you can improve the balance between omega-6 and omega-3 fatty acids, further reducing inflammation.
2. **Improved Lipid Profile**:
   - **Heart Health**: Consuming healthy fats can improve lipid profiles by increasing HDL (good) cholesterol and reducing LDL (bad) cholesterol levels. This supports cardiovascular health, which is closely linked to kidney health.
   - **Metabolic Benefits**: Healthy fats can help regulate blood sugar levels and reduce the risk of insulin resistance and metabolic syndrome, which are risk factors for kidney disease.
3. **Oxidative Stress Reduction**:
   - **Antioxidant Properties**: Fats like olive oil and avocado oil are rich in antioxidants, which help neutralize free radicals and reduce oxidative stress. Lower oxidative stress levels protect kidney cells from damage and support overall kidney function.
   - **Stable Fats**: Using fats that are stable and less prone to oxidation, such as saturated and monounsaturated fats, reduces the intake of harmful oxidized compounds.
4. **Nutrient Absorption**:
   - **Fat-Soluble Vitamins**: Healthy fats enhance the absorption of fat-soluble vitamins (A, D, E, and K) and other fat-soluble nutrients. These vitamins play crucial roles in bone health, immune function, and overall well-being.

- ◦ **Mineral Absorption**: Certain fats can also aid in the absorption of minerals, such as calcium and magnesium, which are important for kidney health.

5. **Satiety and Weight Management**:
   - ◦ **Feeling Full**: Healthy fats contribute to a feeling of fullness and satiety, helping to regulate appetite and reduce overeating. This can support weight management, which is important for reducing the risk of kidney disease and other chronic conditions.
   - ◦ **Energy Source**: Healthy fats provide a steady source of energy, supporting physical activity and overall vitality.

Practical Tips for Incorporating Healthy Fats into Your Diet

1. **Cooking**:
   - ◦ **Use Olive Oil for Low to Medium-Heat Cooking**: Drizzle olive oil over salads, use it in dressings, or cook with it at low to medium heat.
   - ◦ **Coconut Oil for High-Heat Cooking**: Use coconut oil for baking, frying, and high-heat sautéing due to its stability.
   - ◦ **Butter and Ghee for Flavor**: Enhance the flavor of your dishes by cooking with butter or ghee. They are excellent for sautéing vegetables and roasting meats.

2. **Meal Preparation**:
   - ◦ **Avocado Oil for Versatility**: Incorporate avocado oil in dressings, marinades, and as a finishing oil for roasted vegetables and meats.
   - ◦ **Add Nuts and Seeds**: Include healthy nuts and seeds like almonds, chia seeds, and flaxseeds in your meals for additional healthy fats and nutrients.
   - ◦ **Animal Fats for Traditional Cooking**: Use tallow and lard for traditional recipes and high-heat cooking methods.

3. **Snacking**:

- **Healthy Fat Snacks**: Choose snacks that include healthy fats, such as a handful of nuts, guacamole with vegetable sticks, or a small serving of cheese.

4. **Dining Out**:
   - **Request Healthy Fats**: When dining out, ask for your food to be cooked in olive oil or butter instead of seed oils.
   - **Avoid Fried Foods**: Choose grilled, roasted, or steamed options instead of fried foods, which are often cooked in seed oils.

Sample Meal Plan Featuring Healthy Fats
Day 1:

- **Breakfast**:
   - Scrambled eggs cooked in butter with spinach and tomatoes
   - A small serving of avocado slices
- **Lunch**:
   - Grilled chicken salad with mixed greens, cucumbers, bell peppers, and an olive oil-lemon dressing
   - A serving of quinoa
- **Snack**:
   - A handful of almonds
- **Dinner**:
   - Baked salmon with a side of steamed broccoli and roasted sweet potatoes, drizzled with avocado oil
   - A serving of brown rice

Day 2:

- **Breakfast**:
   - Greek yogurt (plain, unsweetened) topped with chia seeds and fresh berries
   - A small bowl of mixed nuts

- **Lunch**:
  - Turkey and avocado wrap using a whole grain tortilla, filled with leafy greens and sliced red bell peppers
  - Carrot sticks with hummus
- **Snack**:
  - Sliced apple with almond butter
- **Dinner**:
  - Roasted chicken thighs with a side of sautéed kale and garlic, cooked in olive oil
  - A serving of wild rice

Conclusion

Avoiding seed oils and incorporating healthy fats into your diet can have significant benefits for kidney health and overall well-being. Seed oils, high in omega-6 fatty acids and prone to oxidation, can promote inflammation and oxidative stress, contributing to kidney damage and other chronic diseases. In contrast, healthy fats from sources like olive oil, coconut oil, avocado oil, butter, and animal fats provide anti-inflammatory properties, support heart health, and enhance nutrient absorption. By choosing stable, nutrient-rich fats and incorporating them into your daily meals, you can protect your kidneys, reduce inflammation, and support overall health.

Chapter 16: Cooking Techniques for Optimal Health
Introduction

Cooking techniques play a crucial role in preserving the nutritional value of foods and minimizing the formation of harmful substances. For individuals with kidney issues, adopting healthy cooking methods is essential to ensure meals are both nutritious and safe. This chapter explores the best cooking methods to preserve nutrients and avoid harmful substances, along with recipes and tips for kidney-friendly cooking.

Best Cooking Methods to Preserve Nutrients and Avoid Harmful Substances

1. **Steaming:**
   - **Nutrient Preservation**: Steaming is one of the best methods for preserving the nutrients in vegetables and proteins. It prevents the loss of water-soluble vitamins and minerals that can occur during boiling.
   - **Minimal Fat Use**: Steaming requires little to no added fat, making it a healthy option for preparing a variety of foods.
   - **How to Steam**: Use a steamer basket over boiling water or a dedicated electric steamer. Steam vegetables until tender but still vibrant in color.

2. **Grilling:**
   - **Flavor and Nutrients**: Grilling adds a smoky flavor to foods without the need for excessive fats or oils. It also helps retain nutrients in meats and vegetables.
   - **Avoid Charring**: To minimize the formation of harmful compounds like heterocyclic amines (HCAs) and

polycyclic aromatic hydrocarbons (PAHs), avoid charring the food. Use lower heat and turn foods frequently.

- **How to Grill**: Preheat the grill to medium heat. Grill meats and vegetables until they reach a safe internal temperature and are cooked to your preference.

3. **Baking**:

- **Healthy and Versatile**: Baking is a versatile cooking method that retains the nutrients in foods while allowing for a variety of preparations, from meats to vegetables to healthy baked goods.
- **Low-Fat Cooking**: Baking typically requires less fat than frying, making it a healthier option.
- **How to Bake**: Preheat the oven to the desired temperature. Use parchment paper or a silicone baking mat to reduce the need for added oils. Bake until foods are cooked through and golden brown.

4. **Roasting**:

- **Enhancing Flavor**: Roasting concentrates the natural flavors of foods and caramelizes their sugars, adding depth to meats and vegetables.
- **Nutrient Retention**: Roasting preserves nutrients while reducing the need for excessive fats.
- **How to Roast**: Preheat the oven to 400°F (200°C). Toss vegetables or meats with a small amount of healthy fat (e.g., olive oil) and seasonings. Roast until tender and caramelized.

5. **Sautéing**:

- **Quick and Nutritious**: Sautéing is a quick cooking method that uses a small amount of fat to cook foods over medium-high heat. It retains the nutrients and flavors of ingredients.
- **Healthy Fats**: Use healthy fats like olive oil, coconut oil, or avocado oil for sautéing.

- ◦ **How to Sauté**: Heat a small amount of oil in a skillet over medium-high heat. Add ingredients and cook, stirring frequently, until tender and cooked through.

6. **Slow Cooking**:
    - ◦ **Nutrient Retention**: Slow cooking at low temperatures preserves nutrients and enhances the flavors of ingredients.
    - ◦ **Convenience**: Slow cookers allow for easy meal preparation, making it convenient to cook nutritious meals.
    - ◦ **How to Slow Cook**: Add ingredients to a slow cooker and set the temperature to low or high, depending on the recipe. Cook for several hours until ingredients are tender and flavors melded.

7. **Poaching**:
    - ◦ **Gentle Cooking**: Poaching involves cooking foods gently in simmering liquid, preserving their nutrients and delicate textures.
    - ◦ **Flavor Infusion**: Poaching liquids can be seasoned with herbs, spices, and aromatics to infuse flavors into the food.
    - ◦ **How to Poach**: Heat a poaching liquid (water, broth, or milk) to a simmer. Add the food and cook gently until done.

Recipes and Tips for Kidney-Friendly Cooking

1. **Grilled Chicken with Lemon and Herbs**

Ingredients:

- 4 boneless, skinless chicken breasts
- 2 tablespoons olive oil
- Juice of 1 lemon
- 2 cloves garlic, minced
- 1 teaspoon dried oregano

- 1 teaspoon dried thyme
- Salt and pepper to taste

Instructions:

1. Preheat the grill to medium heat.
2. In a bowl, combine olive oil, lemon juice, garlic, oregano, thyme, salt, and pepper.
3. Brush the chicken breasts with the marinade and let them sit for 10 minutes.
4. Grill the chicken for 6-7 minutes on each side or until the internal temperature reaches 165°F (74°C).
5. Serve with a side of steamed vegetables or a fresh salad.

Tips:

- Marinating the chicken adds flavor and helps keep it moist during grilling.
- Use a meat thermometer to ensure the chicken is cooked to a safe temperature.

1. **Baked Salmon with Dill and Lemon**

Ingredients:

- 4 salmon fillets
- 2 tablespoons olive oil
- Juice of 1 lemon
- 2 tablespoons fresh dill, chopped
- Salt and pepper to taste

Instructions:

1. Preheat the oven to 375°F (190°C).
2. Place the salmon fillets on a baking sheet lined with parchment paper.
3. Drizzle the olive oil and lemon juice over the salmon. Sprinkle with dill, salt, and pepper.
4. Bake for 15-20 minutes or until the salmon flakes easily with a fork.
5. Serve with a side of roasted vegetables or a quinoa salad.

Tips:

- Baking on parchment paper reduces the need for additional oils and makes cleanup easier.
- Dill and lemon enhance the natural flavors of the salmon without adding extra calories.

1. **Roasted Vegetable Medley**

Ingredients:

- 2 cups broccoli florets
- 2 cups cauliflower florets
- 1 cup baby carrots
- 1 red bell pepper, sliced
- 2 tablespoons olive oil
- 1 teaspoon dried thyme
- 1 teaspoon dried rosemary
- Salt and pepper to taste

Instructions:

1. Preheat the oven to 400°F (200°C).

2. In a large bowl, toss the vegetables with olive oil, thyme, rosemary, salt, and pepper.
3. Spread the vegetables on a baking sheet in a single layer.
4. Roast for 20-25 minutes, stirring halfway through, until the vegetables are tender and caramelized.
5. Serve as a side dish with grilled or baked protein.

Tips:

- Cut vegetables into similar-sized pieces to ensure even cooking.
- Roasting at a high temperature helps to caramelize the vegetables, enhancing their natural sweetness.

1. **Sautéed Spinach with Garlic**

Ingredients:

- 1 tablespoon olive oil
- 2 cloves garlic, minced
- 8 cups fresh spinach leaves
- Salt and pepper to taste
- Juice of 1/2 lemon

Instructions:

1. Heat the olive oil in a large skillet over medium-high heat.
2. Add the garlic and sauté for 1-2 minutes until fragrant.
3. Add the spinach and cook, stirring frequently, until wilted, about 3-4 minutes.
4. Season with salt, pepper, and a squeeze of lemon juice.
5. Serve immediately as a side dish.

Tips:

- Sautéing spinach quickly preserves its bright green color and nutrients.
- Adding lemon juice enhances the flavor and provides a fresh finish.

1. **Slow Cooker Chicken and Vegetable Stew**

Ingredients:

- 4 boneless, skinless chicken thighs, cut into chunks
- 2 cups low-sodium chicken broth
- 1 cup baby carrots
- 2 cups diced potatoes
- 1 cup diced celery
- 1 cup diced onion
- 2 cloves garlic, minced
- 1 teaspoon dried thyme
- 1 teaspoon dried rosemary
- Salt and pepper to taste

Instructions:

1. Place the chicken, broth, carrots, potatoes, celery, onion, and garlic in a slow cooker.
2. Add thyme, rosemary, salt, and pepper.
3. Cover and cook on low for 6-8 hours or on high for 3-4 hours until the chicken is tender and the vegetables are cooked.
4. Serve hot with a side of whole-grain bread.

Tips:

- Using a slow cooker allows for hands-off cooking and tenderizes the chicken and vegetables.

- Adjust the seasoning to your taste and add fresh herbs at the end for extra flavor.

Conclusion

Adopting healthy cooking techniques is essential for preserving the nutritional value of foods and minimizing the formation of harmful substances. Methods such as steaming, grilling, baking, roasting, sautéing, slow cooking, and poaching help retain nutrients while reducing the need for excessive fats and oils. Incorporating these techniques into your daily cooking routine can enhance the flavor and health benefits of your meals, supporting kidney health and overall well-being. Use the provided recipes and tips to create delicious, kidney-friendly dishes that nourish your body and promote optimal health.

Chapter 17: Managing Acid Reflux
Understanding Acid Reflux

Acid reflux, also known as gastroesophageal reflux disease (GERD), occurs when stomach acid flows back into the esophagus, causing symptoms such as heartburn, regurgitation, and discomfort. It can lead to more serious health problems if left untreated. Managing and preventing acid reflux involves dietary changes, lifestyle modifications, and understanding which foods and habits can help alleviate symptoms.

How the Diet Helps Manage and Prevent Acid Reflux

1. **Reducing Acidic Foods**:
   - **Acidic Triggers**: Foods that are high in acidity, such as citrus fruits, tomatoes, and vinegar, can trigger acid reflux symptoms by irritating the esophagus and increasing stomach acid production.
   - **Alkaline Foods**: Incorporating more alkaline foods into the diet can help neutralize stomach acid and reduce reflux symptoms. Alkaline foods, such as leafy greens, cucumbers, and melons, have a higher pH and can help balance the body's acidity.

2. **Avoiding High-Fat Foods**:
   - **Fat and Reflux**: High-fat foods slow down the digestive process and relax the lower esophageal sphincter (LES), which can cause acid to escape into the esophagus. Reducing the intake of fried foods, fatty meats, and full-fat dairy products can help prevent reflux.
   - **Lean Proteins**: Opting for lean proteins, such as chicken, turkey, fish, and plant-based proteins, can reduce the risk

of acid reflux by promoting faster digestion and lessening pressure on the LES.

3. **Eliminating Trigger Foods:**
    ◦ **Common Triggers**: Certain foods and beverages, such as caffeine, alcohol, chocolate, and spicy foods, are known to trigger acid reflux. Eliminating or reducing these triggers from the diet can help manage symptoms.
    ◦ **Trigger Identification**: Keeping a food diary to track what you eat and when you experience symptoms can help identify specific triggers and make it easier to avoid them.
4. **Eating Smaller, More Frequent Meals:**
    ◦ **Portion Control**: Eating large meals can increase stomach pressure and cause the LES to open, leading to reflux. Smaller, more frequent meals can help reduce this pressure and prevent symptoms.
    ◦ **Meal Timing**: Avoid lying down immediately after eating, and aim to finish meals at least three hours before bedtime to allow time for digestion.

Specific Foods and Habits to Incorporate for Relief

1. **Foods to Include:**

- **Non-Citrus Fruits:**
    ◦ **Bananas**: Low in acid and can help coat the esophageal lining, reducing discomfort.
    ◦ **Melons**: Alkaline and hydrating, melons can help neutralize stomach acid.
- **Vegetables:**
    ◦ **Leafy Greens**: Spinach, kale, and other greens are low in fat and acid, making them ideal for managing reflux.
    ◦ **Cucumbers and Celery**: These vegetables are high in water content, which can dilute stomach acid and provide relief.

- **Whole Grains:**
  - **Oatmeal:** High in fiber and low in fat, oatmeal can help absorb stomach acid and reduce reflux.
  - **Brown Rice and Quinoa:** These grains are easy to digest and less likely to cause reflux.
- **Lean Proteins:**
  - **Chicken and Turkey:** Skinless poultry is low in fat and can be easily digested.
  - **Fish:** Non-fatty fish like cod and tilapia are good sources of protein without triggering reflux.
  - **Plant-Based Proteins:** Lentils, chickpeas, and tofu are excellent sources of protein that are less likely to cause reflux.
- **Healthy Fats:**
  - **Avocados:** While higher in fat, avocados contain healthy monounsaturated fats that can be included in moderation.
  - **Nuts and Seeds:** Almonds, flaxseeds, and chia seeds provide healthy fats and fiber.

1. **Foods to Avoid:**

- **Citrus Fruits and Juices:** Oranges, lemons, limes, and grapefruits can increase stomach acidity and trigger reflux.
- **Tomatoes and Tomato Products:** Tomato sauce, ketchup, and other tomato-based products are highly acidic.
- **Chocolate:** Contains caffeine and other compounds that can relax the LES.
- **Spicy Foods:** Hot peppers and spices like chili powder can irritate the esophagus.
- **High-Fat Foods:** Fried foods, fatty meats, and full-fat dairy products slow digestion and increase reflux risk.
- **Caffeine and Alcohol:** Both can relax the LES and increase stomach acid production.

1. **Beneficial Habits:**

- **Chew Thoroughly**: Eating slowly and chewing food thoroughly can aid digestion and reduce the likelihood of reflux.
- **Stay Upright**: Avoid lying down immediately after meals. Stay upright for at least 2-3 hours to allow proper digestion.
- **Elevate the Head of the Bed**: Elevating the head of the bed by about 6-8 inches can help prevent nighttime reflux by keeping stomach acid down.
- **Wear Loose Clothing**: Tight clothing can put pressure on the abdomen and LES, leading to reflux.
- **Weight Management**: Maintaining a healthy weight can reduce abdominal pressure and decrease the risk of reflux.

1. **Hydration:**

- **Water**: Drinking water can help wash down stomach acid and dilute its concentration in the stomach. Aim to drink water throughout the day but avoid large amounts during meals.
- **Herbal Teas**: Ginger tea, chamomile tea, and licorice tea can soothe the digestive system and reduce reflux symptoms.

Sample Meal Plan for Managing Acid Reflux
Day 1:

- **Breakfast:**
    - Oatmeal with sliced bananas and a sprinkle of flaxseeds
    - Herbal tea (ginger tea)
- **Mid-Morning Snack:**
    - A small handful of almonds
- **Lunch:**
    - Grilled chicken salad with mixed greens, cucumbers, bell peppers, and a light olive oil and lemon dressing

- ○ A side of quinoa
- **Afternoon Snack:**
    - ○ Sliced apple with a small serving of almond butter
- **Dinner:**
    - ○ Baked salmon with a side of steamed broccoli and roasted sweet potatoes
    - ○ A serving of brown rice

Day 2:

- **Breakfast:**
    - ○ Smoothie with spinach, cucumber, melon, and chia seeds
    - ○ Herbal tea (chamomile tea)
- **Mid-Morning Snack:**
    - ○ A small bowl of mixed berries
- **Lunch:**
    - ○ Turkey and avocado wrap using a whole grain tortilla, filled with leafy greens and sliced red bell peppers
    - ○ Carrot sticks with hummus
- **Afternoon Snack:**
    - ○ A small serving of plain Greek yogurt with a drizzle of honey and a sprinkle of flaxseeds
- **Dinner:**
    - ○ Roasted chicken thighs with a side of sautéed kale and garlic
    - ○ A serving of wild rice

Conclusion

Managing acid reflux requires a comprehensive approach that includes dietary changes and lifestyle modifications. By avoiding trigger foods, incorporating alkaline and nutrient-rich foods, and adopting healthy eating habits, you can effectively manage and prevent acid reflux symptoms. The provided meal plans and tips offer practical ways to incorporate these changes into your daily routine, supporting both digestive health and overall well-being. Embrace these strategies to enjoy meals without discomfort and promote long-term health.

notes:

Chapter 18: Coping with Dietary Changes

Introduction

Transitioning from a diet filled with junk food to a purer, kidney-friendly diet can be challenging both emotionally and psychologically. Such significant dietary changes require not only physical adjustments but also mental and emotional resilience. This chapter provides support and practical strategies to help you navigate this transition, stay motivated, and manage cravings. Remember, making these changes is a journey, and every step you take towards a healthier diet is a step towards better health and well-being.

Emotional and Psychological Aspects of Transitioning to the Diet

1. **Understanding Emotional Connections to Food:**
   - **Comfort and Stress Eating**: Many people turn to junk food as a source of comfort during stressful times. Recognizing these emotional connections can help you understand why certain foods are appealing and how they affect your mood.
   - **Cultural and Social Influences**: Food is often tied to social gatherings, traditions, and cultural practices. Changing your diet can sometimes feel isolating or challenging when it differs from those around you.

2. **Dealing with Resistance and Frustration:**
   - **Initial Resistance**: It's natural to resist changes, especially when it comes to food preferences and habits. Acknowledge that initial resistance is part of the process and give yourself grace as you adjust.
   - **Frustration and Setbacks**: There will be days when cravings are strong, or you might slip back into old eating

habits. Understand that setbacks are normal and don't mean failure. Each day is a new opportunity to make healthier choices.

3. **Building a Positive Mindset:**
   - **Focus on Benefits**: Remind yourself of the reasons for making these changes, such as improved kidney health, increased energy, and overall well-being. Keeping the benefits in mind can help you stay motivated.
   - **Celebrate Small Wins**: Acknowledge and celebrate small victories, whether it's choosing a healthy snack over junk food or successfully preparing a kidney-friendly meal. Each positive choice is progress.

Tips for Staying Motivated and Managing Cravings

1. **Setting Realistic Goals:**
   - **Short-Term Goals**: Set achievable short-term goals, such as trying a new healthy recipe each week or reducing the number of junk food snacks by one per day.
   - **Long-Term Goals**: Define long-term health goals, like improving kidney function or reaching a healthier weight. Write them down and revisit them regularly to stay focused.

2. **Creating a Support System:**
   - **Family and Friends**: Share your dietary goals with family and friends. Their support can make a significant difference, and they might join you in making healthier choices.
   - **Support Groups**: Consider joining a support group, either in person or online, where you can share experiences, recipes, and encouragement with others on a similar journey.

3. **Planning and Preparation:**

- **Meal Planning**: Plan your meals and snacks in advance to avoid the temptation of junk food. Having healthy options readily available makes it easier to stick to your diet.
- **Grocery Shopping**: Create a shopping list based on your meal plan and stick to it. Avoid aisles that are heavily stocked with junk food to minimize temptation.

4. **Healthy Substitutions**:
   - **Alternative Snacks**: Replace junk food with healthier alternatives. For example, choose air-popped popcorn instead of chips, or fruit and nuts instead of candy.
   - **Creative Cooking**: Experiment with new recipes that use healthier ingredients. You might discover that you enjoy the taste and feel better after eating cleaner foods.

5. **Managing Cravings**:
   - **Understand Cravings**: Cravings are often a sign of hunger, dehydration, or emotional triggers. Address the underlying cause by eating balanced meals, drinking water, or finding stress-relief activities.
   - **Healthy Distractions**: When cravings hit, distract yourself with a healthy activity such as going for a walk, reading a book, or calling a friend. Often, the craving will pass after a few minutes.

6. **Mindful Eating**:
   - **Pay Attention to Hunger Cues**: Eat when you're hungry and stop when you're full. Avoid eating out of boredom or stress.
   - **Enjoy Your Food**: Take time to savor your meals, focusing on the flavors, textures, and aromas. Eating mindfully can enhance your appreciation for healthy foods and reduce the desire for junk food.

7. **Incorporating Treats**:
   - **Moderation**: It's okay to enjoy treats in moderation. Allowing yourself an occasional indulgence can prevent

feelings of deprivation and help you stick to your diet in the long run.

- ◦ **Healthier Treats**: Find ways to make healthier versions of your favorite treats, such as using whole-grain flour, natural sweeteners, or baking instead of frying.

Sample Daily Routine for Staying Motivated
Morning:

- **Hydration**: Start your day with a glass of water with a splash of lemon juice.
- **Healthy Breakfast**: Prepare a nutritious breakfast, such as oatmeal with fresh fruit and nuts.
- **Set Intentions**: Take a few minutes to set your intentions for the day, focusing on making healthy choices.

Mid-Morning:

- **Snack**: Have a small, healthy snack, such as a piece of fruit or a handful of almonds.
- **Activity**: Take a short walk or stretch to boost your energy and mood.

Lunch:

- **Balanced Meal**: Enjoy a balanced lunch with lean protein, whole grains, and plenty of vegetables.
- **Social Connection**: Connect with a friend or colleague to share your progress and stay motivated.

Afternoon:

- **Hydration**: Drink water or herbal tea to stay hydrated.

- **Snack**: Choose a healthy snack, such as yogurt with berries or sliced vegetables with hummus.

Dinner:

- **Nutritious Dinner**: Prepare a kidney-friendly dinner, such as baked salmon with roasted vegetables and quinoa.
- **Relaxation**: Spend time relaxing and engaging in activities that bring you joy, such as reading, hobbies, or spending time with loved ones.

Evening:

- **Reflection**: Reflect on your day and acknowledge your successes, no matter how small.
- **Planning**: Plan your meals and activities for the next day to stay on track.

Encouragement and Support

1. **Be Kind to Yourself**:
   - **Self-Compassion**: Practice self-compassion and be kind to yourself during this transition. Understand that making significant dietary changes takes time and effort.
   - **Positive Self-Talk**: Replace negative thoughts with positive affirmations. Remind yourself of your strengths and the progress you've made.
2. **Stay Inspired**:
   - **Success Stories**: Read success stories of others who have made similar dietary changes. Their experiences can inspire and motivate you to keep going.

- **Educational Resources**: Educate yourself about the benefits of a healthy diet for kidney health and overall well-being. Knowledge can empower you to make informed choices.

3. **Reward Yourself**:
   - **Non-Food Rewards**: Reward yourself for reaching milestones with non-food treats, such as a new book, a relaxing bath, or a fun outing.
   - **Celebrate Progress**: Celebrate your progress and achievements, no matter how small. Each step towards a healthier diet is a victory.

Conclusion

Transitioning to a purer, kidney-friendly diet can be challenging, but it's a journey worth taking for your health and well-being. By understanding the emotional and psychological aspects of dietary changes, setting realistic goals, and creating a support system, you can navigate this transition with confidence. Use the tips for staying motivated and managing cravings to make the process smoother and more enjoyable. Remember, every healthy choice you make brings you closer to a healthier, happier life. Embrace the journey and celebrate your progress along the way.

Chapter 19: Seasonal and Holiday Eating

Introduction

Holidays and special occasions often revolve around food, making it challenging to maintain a kidney-friendly diet during these times. However, with careful planning and the right strategies, you can enjoy festive meals while adhering to your dietary goals. This chapter offers practical tips for navigating seasonal and holiday eating and provides kidney-friendly recipes and meal ideas to help you stay on track.

Strategies for Maintaining the Diet During Holidays and Special Occasions

1. **Plan Ahead:**
   - **Menu Planning**: Plan your holiday menu in advance to ensure it includes kidney-friendly options. This allows you to make healthier choices and avoid last-minute temptations.
   - **Bring Your Own Dish**: If attending a gathering, offer to bring a kidney-friendly dish. This ensures there will be something you can eat and share with others.
2. **Modify Traditional Recipes:**
   - **Healthier Substitutions**: Modify traditional holiday recipes to make them kidney-friendly. Use lean proteins, reduce sodium, and incorporate plenty of vegetables.
   - **Portion Control**: Enjoy smaller portions of higher-calorie or less healthy dishes. This allows you to partake in the celebration without overindulging.
3. **Stay Hydrated:**
   - **Drink Water**: Drink plenty of water throughout the day to stay hydrated and support kidney function. Avoid sugary

drinks and alcohol, which can dehydrate you and worsen kidney issues.

- ◦ **Herbal Teas**: Enjoy herbal teas like ginger tea or chamomile tea as festive, kidney-friendly beverages.

4. **Mindful Eating**:
   - ◦ **Eat Slowly**: Take your time to savor each bite, which can help you feel more satisfied and prevent overeating.
   - ◦ **Listen to Your Body**: Pay attention to hunger and fullness cues. Eat when you're hungry and stop when you're satisfied.

5. **Focus on Socializing**:
   - ◦ **Engage in Conversations**: Focus on socializing and enjoying the company of family and friends. This can take the emphasis off food and make the event more enjoyable.
   - ◦ **Activities and Traditions**: Participate in non-food-related holiday activities and traditions, such as playing games, going for a walk, or engaging in festive crafts.

6. **Set Realistic Expectations**:
   - ◦ **Be Flexible**: Understand that it's okay to indulge occasionally, but aim to make the majority of your choices kidney-friendly.
   - ◦ **Forgive Slip-Ups**: If you do indulge more than planned, don't be too hard on yourself. Get back on track with your next meal and focus on long-term consistency.

Kidney-Friendly Holiday Recipes and Meal Ideas

1. **Appetizers**:

- **Stuffed Mushrooms**:

Ingredients:

- 16 large button mushrooms
- 1 tablespoon olive oil
- 1 small onion, finely chopped
- 2 cloves garlic, minced
- 1/2 cup whole-wheat breadcrumbs
- 1/4 cup grated Parmesan cheese
- 2 tablespoons fresh parsley, chopped
- Salt and pepper to taste

Instructions:

1. Preheat the oven to 375°F (190°C).
2. Remove the stems from the mushrooms and finely chop them.
3. Heat olive oil in a skillet over medium heat. Sauté the onion, garlic, and chopped mushroom stems until softened.
4. In a bowl, combine the sautéed vegetables, breadcrumbs, Parmesan cheese, parsley, salt, and pepper.
5. Stuff the mushroom caps with the mixture and place them on a baking sheet.
6. Bake for 15-20 minutes or until the mushrooms are tender and the filling is golden brown.

- **Vegetable Platter with Hummus:**

Ingredients:

- Assorted fresh vegetables (carrots, celery, bell peppers, cucumber, cherry tomatoes)
- 1 cup hummus (store-bought or homemade)

Instructions:

1. Wash and cut the vegetables into bite-sized pieces.

2. Arrange the vegetables on a platter and serve with hummus for dipping.
3. **Main Courses:**

• **Herb-Roasted Turkey:**

Ingredients:

- 1 whole turkey (10-12 pounds), thawed if frozen
- 1/4 cup olive oil
- 2 tablespoons fresh rosemary, chopped
- 2 tablespoons fresh thyme, chopped
- 2 tablespoons fresh sage, chopped
- 1 lemon, sliced
- 1 onion, quartered
- 4 cloves garlic, smashed
- Salt and pepper to taste

Instructions:

1. Preheat the oven to 325°F (165°C).
2. In a small bowl, combine olive oil, rosemary, thyme, sage, salt, and pepper.
3. Rub the herb mixture all over the turkey, including under the skin.
4. Stuff the cavity with lemon slices, onion quarters, and garlic cloves.
5. Place the turkey on a rack in a roasting pan and roast for 3-4 hours, or until the internal temperature reaches 165°F (74°C). Baste occasionally with pan juices.
6. Let the turkey rest for 20 minutes before carving.

• **Baked Salmon with Dill and Lemon:**

Ingredients:

- 4 salmon fillets
- 2 tablespoons olive oil
- Juice of 1 lemon
- 2 tablespoons fresh dill, chopped
- Salt and pepper to taste

Instructions:

1. Preheat the oven to 375°F (190°C).
2. Place the salmon fillets on a baking sheet lined with parchment paper.
3. Drizzle the olive oil and lemon juice over the salmon. Sprinkle with dill, salt, and pepper.
4. Bake for 15-20 minutes or until the salmon flakes easily with a fork.
5. Serve with a side of steamed vegetables or a quinoa salad.
6. **Side Dishes:**

- **Roasted Vegetable Medley:**

Ingredients:

- 2 cups broccoli florets
- 2 cups cauliflower florets
- 1 cup baby carrots
- 1 red bell pepper, sliced
- 2 tablespoons olive oil
- 1 teaspoon dried thyme
- 1 teaspoon dried rosemary
- Salt and pepper to taste

Instructions:

1. Preheat the oven to 400°F (200°C).
2. In a large bowl, toss the vegetables with olive oil, thyme, rosemary, salt, and pepper.
3. Spread the vegetables on a baking sheet in a single layer.
4. Roast for 20-25 minutes, stirring halfway through, until the vegetables are tender and caramelized.
5. Serve as a side dish with grilled or baked protein.

- **Quinoa Salad with Cranberries and Almonds:**

Ingredients:

- 1 cup quinoa, rinsed
- 2 cups low-sodium chicken broth or water
- 1/2 cup dried cranberries
- 1/2 cup sliced almonds, toasted
- 2 green onions, sliced
- 1/4 cup fresh parsley, chopped
- 2 tablespoons olive oil
- Juice of 1 lemon
- Salt and pepper to taste

Instructions:

1. In a medium saucepan, bring the chicken broth or water to a boil. Add the quinoa, reduce heat, cover, and simmer for 15 minutes or until the liquid is absorbed.
2. Remove from heat and let the quinoa cool.
3. In a large bowl, combine the cooled quinoa, cranberries, almonds, green onions, and parsley.

4. In a small bowl, whisk together the olive oil, lemon juice, salt, and pepper. Pour over the quinoa mixture and toss to combine.
5. Serve as a side dish or light main course.
6. **Desserts:**

- **Baked Apples with Cinnamon:**

Ingredients:

- 4 large apples
- 1/4 cup rolled oats
- 2 tablespoons chopped walnuts
- 2 tablespoons honey
- 1 teaspoon ground cinnamon
- 1/4 teaspoon ground nutmeg
- 1/4 cup water

Instructions:

1. Preheat the oven to 350°F (175°C).
2. Core the apples and place them in a baking dish.
3. In a small bowl, combine the oats, walnuts, honey, cinnamon, and nutmeg. Stuff the mixture into the cored apples.
4. Pour the water into the baking dish around the apples.
5. Bake for 30-35 minutes, or until the apples are tender.
6. Serve warm, optionally with a dollop of plain Greek yogurt.

Conclusion

Holidays and special occasions don't have to derail your kidney-friendly diet. By planning ahead, modifying traditional recipes, and focusing on mindful eating, you can enjoy festive meals without compromising your health. The provided strategies and recipes offer delicious, kidney-friendly alternatives that will help you stay on track and celebrate with confidence. Embrace these tips to make your holidays both enjoyable and healthful, and remember that each positive choice contributes to your long-term well-being.

Chapter 20: Meal Planning and Preparation

Introduction

Effective meal planning and preparation are essential components of maintaining a kidney-friendly diet. By planning your meals in advance, you can ensure that you're meeting your nutritional needs, saving time and money, and avoiding unhealthy food choices. This chapter provides practical advice for meal planning and preparation, including sample meal plans and grocery lists to help you stay organized and committed to your dietary goals.

Practical Advice for Planning and Preparing Meals

1. **Set Clear Goals:**
   - **Dietary Objectives:** Define your dietary objectives based on your kidney health needs, such as reducing sodium intake, increasing hydration, or balancing protein consumption.
   - **Weekly Planning:** Plan your meals on a weekly basis to ensure variety and balance in your diet. This helps prevent repetitive eating and ensures you get a wide range of nutrients.

2. **Create a Meal Plan:**
   - **Balanced Meals:** Ensure each meal includes a balance of lean proteins, healthy fats, vegetables, and whole grains. This supports overall health and kidney function.
   - **Meal Variety:** Rotate different types of proteins, vegetables, and grains throughout the week to keep meals interesting and nutritionally diverse.

3. **Organize Your Grocery Shopping:**

- **Make a List**: Create a detailed grocery list based on your meal plan. This helps you avoid impulse purchases and ensures you have all the ingredients you need.
- **Shop Smart**: Stick to the perimeter of the grocery store where fresh produce, meats, and dairy are typically located. Avoid the aisles with processed and packaged foods.

4. **Prepare Ingredients in Advance**:
   - **Batch Cooking**: Prepare larger batches of staple ingredients like grains, proteins, and vegetables. This saves time and makes it easier to assemble meals during the week.
   - **Pre-Chop Vegetables**: Wash and chop vegetables in advance to reduce meal preparation time. Store them in airtight containers in the refrigerator.

5. **Utilize Kitchen Tools**:
   - **Slow Cooker and Instant Pot**: These appliances can simplify meal preparation by allowing you to cook large batches of food with minimal effort.
   - **Storage Containers**: Invest in quality storage containers to keep prepped ingredients fresh and organized.

6. **Incorporate Leftovers**:
   - **Plan for Leftovers**: Cook extra portions for dinner to have leftovers for lunch the next day. This reduces the need for additional meal preparation.
   - **Creative Repurposing**: Repurpose leftovers into new meals. For example, use leftover roasted vegetables in a salad or grain bowl.

Sample Meal Plans and Grocery Lists
Sample Meal Plan for One Week
Day 1:

- **Breakfast**: Greek yogurt with fresh berries and a sprinkle of chia seeds

- **Lunch**: Grilled chicken salad with mixed greens, cucumbers, bell peppers, and a lemon-tahini dressing
- **Snack**: Sliced apple with almond butter
- **Dinner**: Baked salmon with steamed broccoli and quinoa

Day 2:

- **Breakfast**: Smoothie with spinach, banana, almond milk, and flaxseeds
- **Lunch**: Turkey and avocado wrap using a whole grain tortilla, with a side of carrot sticks and hummus
- **Snack**: A handful of almonds
- **Dinner**: Roasted chicken thighs with sautéed kale and garlic, served with brown rice

Day 3:

- **Breakfast**: Oatmeal topped with sliced banana, walnuts, and a drizzle of honey
- **Lunch**: Quinoa salad with chickpeas, cherry tomatoes, cucumber, and olive oil dressing
- **Snack**: Celery sticks with hummus
- **Dinner**: Grilled tilapia with a side of roasted Brussels sprouts and sweet potato

Day 4:

- **Breakfast**: Scrambled eggs with spinach and tomatoes
- **Lunch**: Lentil soup with a side of whole grain bread
- **Snack**: A small bowl of mixed berries
- **Dinner**: Baked cod with a side of steamed green beans and wild rice

Day 5:

- **Breakfast**: Smoothie bowl with kale, pineapple, almond milk, and chia seeds
- **Lunch**: Grilled chicken Caesar salad with a light dressing
- **Snack**: Sliced bell peppers with guacamole
- **Dinner**: Turkey meatballs with spaghetti squash and marinara sauce

Day 6:

- **Breakfast**: Greek yogurt with granola and fresh strawberries
- **Lunch**: Vegetable stir-fry with tofu and brown rice
- **Snack**: A handful of cashews
- **Dinner**: Roasted pork tenderloin with a side of roasted carrots and quinoa

Day 7:

- **Breakfast**: Overnight oats with almond milk, chia seeds, and blueberries
- **Lunch**: Spinach and feta stuffed chicken breast with a side of mixed greens
- **Snack**: A small piece of dark chocolate with a few walnuts
- **Dinner**: Grilled shrimp skewers with a side of grilled vegetables and couscous

Grocery List for One Week
Proteins:

- Chicken breasts (4)
- Salmon fillets (4)
- Turkey breast (1 lb)

- Chicken thighs (4)
- Tilapia fillets (4)
- Cod fillets (4)
- Ground turkey (1 lb)
- Pork tenderloin (1)
- Tofu (1 block)
- Shrimp (1 lb)

Dairy and Alternatives:

- Greek yogurt (32 oz)
- Almond milk (1 quart)
- Feta cheese (4 oz)

Grains and Legumes:

- Quinoa (1 lb)
- Brown rice (1 lb)
- Whole grain tortillas (1 pack)
- Whole grain bread (1 loaf)
- Oatmeal (1 lb)
- Lentils (1 lb)
- Spaghetti squash (1)
- Couscous (1 lb)

Fruits and Vegetables:

- Spinach (1 lb)
- Kale (1 lb)
- Mixed greens (1 lb)
- Cucumbers (4)
- Bell peppers (6)
- Cherry tomatoes (1 pint)

- Carrots (1 lb)
- Sweet potatoes (4)
- Broccoli (2 heads)
- Brussels sprouts (1 lb)
- Green beans (1 lb)
- Apples (6)
- Bananas (6)
- Berries (1 pint each of strawberries, blueberries, raspberries)
- Pineapple (1)
- Avocado (4)
- Lemon (4)
- Garlic (1 bulb)
- Onion (2)

Nuts and Seeds:

- Chia seeds (1 cup)
- Flaxseeds (1 cup)
- Walnuts (1 cup)
- Almonds (1 cup)
- Cashews (1 cup)

Pantry Staples:

- Olive oil (1 bottle)
- Tahini (1 jar)
- Hummus (1 container)
- Low-sodium chicken broth (4 cups)
- Canned chickpeas (2 cans)
- Marinara sauce (1 jar)
- Spices (salt, pepper, thyme, rosemary, cinnamon, nutmeg)

Conclusion

Meal planning and preparation are key components of maintaining a kidney-friendly diet. By setting clear goals, creating balanced meal plans, organizing your grocery shopping, and preparing ingredients in advance, you can make healthy eating more manageable and sustainable. The sample meal plans and grocery lists provided in this chapter offer practical guidance to help you get started. Embrace these strategies to stay organized, save time, and ensure that your diet supports your kidney health and overall well-being.

Author's Note: Adjust this as you feel, Diary may harm your kidney's or other things from this list might, just adjust it as your see fit. Please be safe out there.

Chapter 21: Monitoring and Adjusting the Diet
Introduction

Maintaining a kidney-friendly diet is a dynamic process that requires ongoing monitoring and adjustments to ensure optimal health outcomes. This chapter explores how to effectively monitor kidney health, make necessary dietary adjustments, and the importance of regular check-ups and tracking progress.

How to Monitor Kidney Health and Adjust the Diet

1. **Understanding Key Indicators of Kidney Health:**
   - **Glomerular Filtration Rate (GFR):** GFR measures how well your kidneys filter blood. A lower GFR indicates reduced kidney function. Monitoring GFR regularly helps assess the effectiveness of dietary changes.
   - **Blood Pressure:** High blood pressure can damage the kidneys. Maintaining a healthy blood pressure is crucial for kidney health.
   - **Urine Tests:** Regular urine tests can detect abnormalities such as proteinuria (excess protein in urine), which indicates kidney damage.
   - **Blood Tests:** Blood tests for creatinine and blood urea nitrogen (BUN) levels provide information about kidney function and waste removal efficiency.
2. **Adjusting the Diet Based on Health Indicators:**
   - **Protein Intake:** Adjust protein intake based on GFR and other kidney function tests. Lower protein intake may be necessary for advanced kidney disease, while moderate intake is suitable for early stages.
   - **Sodium Reduction:** Monitor and reduce sodium intake to manage blood pressure and prevent fluid retention. Aim

for less than 2,300 mg per day or as recommended by your healthcare provider.

- **Potassium and Phosphorus Management**: Adjust dietary potassium and phosphorus based on blood test results. High levels of these minerals can be harmful in kidney disease.
- **Hydration**: Ensure adequate hydration to support kidney function, but avoid overhydration which can strain the kidneys. Monitor fluid intake based on individual needs and kidney function.

3. **Using a Food Diary**:
- **Track Intake**: Keep a detailed food diary to track daily intake of proteins, fats, carbohydrates, sodium, potassium, and phosphorus. This helps identify dietary patterns and areas for adjustment.
- **Identify Triggers**: Use the diary to identify foods that may trigger symptoms such as bloating, swelling, or changes in urine output. Adjust the diet to avoid these triggers.
- **Monitor Symptoms**: Record any symptoms related to kidney health, such as changes in energy levels, appetite, or digestion. This information is valuable for your healthcare provider.

4. **Regular Self-Assessment**:
- **Weight Monitoring**: Regularly monitor your weight to detect fluid retention or loss. Sudden changes in weight can indicate issues with kidney function or fluid balance.
- **Blood Pressure Checks**: Check blood pressure regularly at home to ensure it remains within a healthy range. High blood pressure should be addressed promptly.
- **Physical Activity**: Maintain a regular exercise routine that supports cardiovascular health and overall well-being. Adjust the intensity and duration of exercise based on energy levels and kidney health.

Importance of Regular Check-Ups and Tracking Progress

1. **Regular Medical Check-Ups:**
   - **Kidney Function Tests**: Schedule regular check-ups with your healthcare provider to monitor kidney function through blood and urine tests. These tests help assess the effectiveness of your diet and detect any changes in kidney health.
   - **Medication Management**: Review medications regularly with your healthcare provider to ensure they are appropriate for your kidney health. Adjustments may be needed based on test results and dietary changes.
   - **Nutritional Counseling**: Consider regular consultations with a registered dietitian specializing in kidney health. They can provide personalized dietary recommendations and help adjust your meal plan as needed.

2. **Tracking Progress:**
   - **Setting Goals**: Set specific, measurable goals for kidney health, such as achieving a target GFR or reducing blood pressure. Clear goals provide direction and motivation.
   - **Monitoring Changes**: Track changes in key health indicators, such as GFR, blood pressure, weight, and lab results. Use this information to adjust your diet and lifestyle.
   - **Evaluating Dietary Impact**: Assess the impact of dietary changes on your overall health and kidney function. Positive changes should be continued, while adjustments may be needed for any negative effects.

3. **Using Technology:**
   - **Health Apps**: Utilize health apps to track dietary intake, physical activity, and health indicators. Many apps allow you to log food intake, monitor nutrient levels, and set reminders for medications and check-ups.

○ **Wearable Devices**: Consider using wearable devices to monitor physical activity, heart rate, and other health metrics. These devices provide valuable data for managing overall health and kidney function.

Sample Monitoring Schedule
Daily:

- Track food and fluid intake in a food diary.
- Monitor weight and blood pressure.
- Record any symptoms or changes in health.

Weekly:

- Review food diary entries and identify patterns or triggers.
- Adjust meal plans based on dietary needs and health indicators.
- Engage in regular physical activity and log exercise sessions.

Monthly:

- Check blood pressure with a home monitor and log results.
- Assess progress towards health goals and make necessary adjustments.
- Schedule a consultation with a dietitian if needed.

Every 3-6 Months:

- Schedule a check-up with your healthcare provider for blood and urine tests.
- Review and adjust medications as needed.
- Discuss progress and any concerns with your healthcare team.

Tips for Effective Monitoring and Adjustment

1. **Be Consistent**:
   - Consistency is key to effective monitoring. Regularly track health indicators and dietary intake to ensure accurate assessment and timely adjustments.
2. **Stay Informed**:
   - Educate yourself about kidney health and the impact of diet on kidney function. Understanding the rationale behind dietary recommendations can help you stay motivated and compliant.
3. **Communicate with Your Healthcare Team**:
   - Maintain open communication with your healthcare team. Share your food diary, health indicators, and any concerns. Collaborative care ensures comprehensive management of your kidney health.
4. **Adjust Gradually**:
   - Make dietary adjustments gradually to allow your body to adapt. Sudden changes can be overwhelming and difficult to sustain.
5. **Seek Support**:
   - Join support groups or connect with others who are managing kidney health through diet. Sharing experiences and tips can provide encouragement and motivation.

Conclusion

Monitoring and adjusting your diet is a continuous process that requires diligence and commitment. By regularly assessing kidney health indicators, maintaining open communication with your healthcare team, and making informed dietary adjustments, you can effectively manage your kidney health. Use the strategies and tips provided in this chapter to stay proactive and empowered in your journey towards optimal kidney health. Remember, consistent monitoring and adjustments are key to maintaining long-term health and well-being.

Chapter 22: Benefits Beyond Kidney Health

Introduction

While the primary focus of the kidney-friendly diet is to support and improve kidney health, the benefits extend far beyond just the kidneys. Adopting this diet can lead to significant improvements in overall health, including enhanced energy levels, better weight management, and reduced risk of chronic diseases. In this chapter, we explore the additional health benefits of the kidney-friendly diet and share personal testimonies and success stories to inspire and motivate you on your journey.

Additional Health Benefits of the Kidney-Friendly Diet

1. **Improved Energy Levels:**
   - **Balanced Nutrition**: A kidney-friendly diet emphasizes balanced meals with lean proteins, healthy fats, and complex carbohydrates. This balance provides sustained energy throughout the day, preventing energy crashes associated with high-sugar and high-fat diets.
   - **Reduced Toxins**: By eliminating processed foods and incorporating more whole foods, the diet reduces the intake of toxins and artificial additives that can cause fatigue and sluggishness.

2. **Weight Management:**
   - **Lower Caloric Intake**: Focusing on nutrient-dense foods rather than calorie-dense junk foods helps reduce overall caloric intake. This can lead to natural and sustainable weight loss.
   - **Healthy Fats and Proteins**: Incorporating healthy fats and lean proteins helps maintain muscle mass and promotes fat loss. These nutrients also enhance satiety, reducing the likelihood of overeating.

3. **Heart Health:**
   - **Reduced Sodium**: Lowering sodium intake helps manage blood pressure, reducing the risk of hypertension and related cardiovascular diseases.
   - **Healthy Fats**: The diet emphasizes sources of healthy fats, such as avocados, nuts, seeds, and fatty fish, which are beneficial for heart health. These fats help reduce LDL cholesterol levels and increase HDL cholesterol.

4. **Digestive Health:**
   - **High Fiber**: Increased consumption of fruits, vegetables, and whole grains provides ample dietary fiber, promoting regular bowel movements and a healthy digestive system.
   - **Probiotics**: Incorporating probiotic-rich foods like yogurt and kefir supports gut health by maintaining a balanced microbiome, which is crucial for overall well-being.

5. **Anti-Inflammatory Effects:**
   - **Whole Foods**: The diet's focus on whole foods, including fruits, vegetables, nuts, and lean proteins, helps reduce systemic inflammation. Chronic inflammation is a root cause of many diseases, including arthritis, diabetes, and heart disease.
   - **Omega-3 Fatty Acids**: Consuming fatty fish and other sources of omega-3 fatty acids provides potent anti-inflammatory benefits.

6. **Mental Health:**
   - **Stable Blood Sugar Levels**: By avoiding refined sugars and high-glycemic foods, the diet helps maintain stable blood sugar levels, reducing mood swings and improving mental clarity.
   - **Nutrient-Rich Foods**: Nutrient-dense foods provide essential vitamins and minerals that support brain health and cognitive function, potentially reducing the risk of depression and anxiety.

7. **Skin Health**:
    ◦ **Hydration**: Proper hydration and the elimination of dehydrating beverages like soda and alcohol contribute to better skin hydration and appearance.
    ◦ **Antioxidants**: Fruits and vegetables are rich in antioxidants, which protect the skin from oxidative stress and promote a youthful appearance.

Personal Testimonies and Success Stories

1. **Anna's Journey to Better Kidney Health**:
    ◦ **Background**: Anna was diagnosed with stage 3 chronic kidney disease and struggled with fatigue, swelling, and high blood pressure.
    ◦ **Dietary Changes**: With the guidance of a dietitian, Anna adopted the kidney-friendly diet, focusing on reducing sodium, increasing water intake, and incorporating more fruits and vegetables.
    ◦ **Results**: Within six months, Anna experienced significant improvements in her kidney function tests, reduced swelling, and stabilized blood pressure. She also reported higher energy levels and a greater sense of well-being.
2. **John's Weight Loss Success**:
    ◦ **Background**: John had been overweight for most of his adult life and was recently diagnosed with early-stage kidney disease. His doctor recommended weight loss to help manage his condition.
    ◦ **Dietary Changes**: John committed to the kidney-friendly diet, emphasizing lean proteins, whole grains, and healthy fats. He also eliminated sugary drinks and processed foods.
    ◦ **Results**: Over the course of a year, John lost 50 pounds and saw improvements in his kidney function. He also

reported increased stamina, better sleep, and improved mental clarity.

3. **Maria's Enhanced Energy and Heart Health:**
   - **Background:** Maria, a busy professional, struggled with low energy levels and borderline high blood pressure. Concerned about her family history of heart disease, she decided to make a change.
   - **Dietary Changes:** Maria adopted the kidney-friendly diet, focusing on nutrient-dense foods, reducing sodium, and increasing her intake of omega-3 fatty acids through fatty fish and flaxseeds.
   - **Results:** Within three months, Maria's blood pressure normalized, and she felt more energetic and focused. She also noticed improvements in her cholesterol levels and overall cardiovascular health.

4. **David's Battle with Inflammation:**
   - **Background:** David suffered from chronic joint pain due to inflammation. Traditional treatments provided limited relief, so he looked for dietary solutions.
   - **Dietary Changes:** David followed the kidney-friendly diet, incorporating anti-inflammatory foods like leafy greens, berries, and fatty fish while avoiding processed and inflammatory foods.
   - **Results:** David experienced a significant reduction in joint pain and inflammation. His overall health improved, and he found it easier to stay active and enjoy physical activities.

5. **Emily's Mental Health Transformation:**
   - **Background:** Emily struggled with anxiety and mood swings, which affected her daily life and relationships.
   - **Dietary Changes:** Emily adopted the kidney-friendly diet, focusing on whole foods, stable blood sugar levels, and avoiding caffeine and refined sugars.

- ° **Results**: Emily's anxiety levels decreased, and her mood stabilized. She reported better mental clarity and an overall sense of calm and well-being.

Conclusion

The kidney-friendly diet offers a multitude of benefits that extend far beyond kidney health. Improved energy levels, effective weight management, enhanced heart health, better digestion, reduced inflammation, and improved mental and skin health are just a few of the positive outcomes reported by those who have adopted this diet. The personal testimonies and success stories shared in this chapter highlight the transformative potential of the kidney-friendly diet. By embracing these dietary principles, you can achieve not only better kidney health but also a higher quality of life overall. Stay committed to your journey, and remember that each positive change you make brings you closer to optimal health and well-being.

Chapter 23: Addressing Common Challenges

Introduction

Transitioning to and maintaining a kidney-friendly diet can come with a variety of challenges. These challenges can range from dealing with cravings and social situations to managing time and finding appropriate resources. This chapter provides practical solutions to common challenges and highlights the importance of community support and resources to help you succeed on your dietary journey.

Solutions to Common Challenges

1. **Dealing with Cravings**:
   - **Understand the Cravings**: Recognize that cravings, especially for sugar and high-fat foods, are natural and often driven by emotional or physical triggers.
   - **Healthy Alternatives**: Find healthier alternatives to satisfy cravings. For example, if you crave something sweet, reach for fruit like berries or a small piece of dark chocolate. For salty cravings, try air-popped popcorn or roasted chickpeas.
   - **Stay Hydrated**: Sometimes cravings can be a sign of dehydration. Drinking water or herbal tea can help reduce the intensity of cravings.
   - **Balanced Meals**: Ensure your meals are balanced with adequate protein, healthy fats, and fiber to keep you fuller longer and reduce the likelihood of cravings.

2. **Social Situations and Eating Out**:
   - **Plan Ahead**: Look at restaurant menus online before going out to identify kidney-friendly options. Many restaurants

offer healthier choices that can be customized to fit your diet.

- **Communicate Your Needs**: Don't hesitate to communicate your dietary needs to friends, family, or restaurant staff. Most people are understanding and supportive when they know your dietary restrictions are for health reasons.
- **Bring Your Own Dish**: When attending social gatherings, offer to bring a kidney-friendly dish. This ensures you have something to eat and introduces others to your healthy choices.
- **Portion Control**: Practice portion control when eating out. Consider sharing a meal or asking for a to-go box to save half of your meal for later.

3. **Time Management and Meal Preparation**:
   - **Meal Prep**: Dedicate a day each week to meal prep. Prepare and portion out meals for the week to save time and ensure you have healthy options readily available.
   - **Batch Cooking**: Cook larger quantities of staple foods like grains, proteins, and vegetables that can be used in various meals throughout the week.
   - **Simple Recipes**: Use simple, quick recipes that require minimal ingredients and preparation time. Keep a list of go-to recipes that you can prepare on busy days.
   - **Healthy Snacks**: Keep healthy snacks, such as nuts, fruits, and cut vegetables, readily available for quick, on-the-go options.

4. **Staying Motivated**:
   - **Set Realistic Goals**: Set achievable short-term and long-term goals. Celebrate small victories to stay motivated.
   - **Track Progress**: Keep a food diary and monitor your progress. Seeing improvements in your health, energy levels, and well-being can be a powerful motivator.

- **Visual Reminders**: Use visual reminders, such as a vision board or health tracker app, to keep your goals and progress visible.
- **Find Enjoyment**: Discover new, enjoyable recipes and foods within the kidney-friendly diet. Making mealtime fun and exciting can help maintain motivation.

5. **Managing Dietary Restrictions**:
- **Ingredient Substitutions**: Learn about healthy ingredient substitutions that fit within your dietary restrictions. For example, use zucchini noodles instead of pasta or cauliflower rice instead of regular rice.
- **Read Labels**: Be diligent about reading food labels to avoid hidden sodium, phosphorus, and potassium. Opt for whole, unprocessed foods when possible.
- **Variety in Meals**: Avoid monotony by incorporating a variety of foods and recipes. Experiment with different spices, herbs, and cooking methods to keep meals interesting.

6. **Financial Considerations**:
- **Budget-Friendly Foods**: Focus on budget-friendly kidney-friendly foods like beans, lentils, eggs, and seasonal vegetables. Buying in bulk can also help reduce costs.
- **Meal Planning**: Plan meals based on sales and seasonal produce. This can help you make the most of your budget while still eating healthily.
- **Minimize Waste**: Use leftovers creatively to minimize food waste. For example, use leftover vegetables in soups or stir-fries.

Community Support and Resources

1. **Online Communities and Forums**:
- **Social Media Groups**: Join social media groups focused on kidney health and kidney-friendly diets. These groups

can provide support, inspiration, and practical tips from others who are on a similar journey.

- **Online Forums**: Participate in online forums where you can ask questions, share experiences, and receive advice from others managing kidney health through diet.

2. **Local Support Groups:**

- **Kidney Health Organizations**: Many kidney health organizations offer local support groups where you can connect with others, attend educational workshops, and access resources.
- **Community Centers**: Check with local community centers for health and wellness programs that include support for dietary changes and kidney health.

3. **Healthcare Professionals:**

- **Dietitians and Nutritionists**: Work with a registered dietitian or nutritionist who specializes in kidney health. They can provide personalized dietary guidance and help you navigate challenges.
- **Healthcare Providers**: Regular check-ins with your healthcare provider can help monitor your kidney health and adjust your diet as needed. They can also provide referrals to other professionals and resources.

4. **Educational Resources:**

- **Books and Cookbooks**: Invest in cookbooks and educational books focused on kidney-friendly diets. These can provide recipes, meal plans, and in-depth information about managing kidney health through diet.
- **Websites and Blogs**: Follow reputable websites and blogs that offer information, recipes, and tips for maintaining a kidney-friendly diet. Many of these resources are written by healthcare professionals and individuals who have successfully managed kidney health.

5. **Meal Planning Apps:**

- ◦ **Nutrition Tracking**: Use meal planning and nutrition tracking apps to help you stay organized, monitor your intake, and ensure you're meeting your dietary goals.
- ◦ **Recipe Ideas**: Many apps offer recipe suggestions and meal planning tools that can simplify the process of maintaining a kidney-friendly diet.

Sample Support Resources

1. **National Kidney Foundation (NKF)**:
   - ◦ **Website**: www.kidney.org
   - ◦ **Resources**: Educational materials, support groups, diet tips, and webinars.
2. **American Association of Kidney Patients (AAKP)**:
   - ◦ **Website**: www.aakp.org
   - ◦ **Resources**: Patient advocacy, educational events, support groups, and dietary guidelines.
3. **DaVita Kidney Care**:
   - ◦ **Website**: www.davita.com
   - ◦ **Resources**: Kidney-friendly recipes, nutrition tips, and online community support.
4. **Renal Support Network (RSN)**:
   - ◦ **Website**: www.rsnhope.org
   - ◦ **Resources**: Support groups, educational resources, and patient stories.

Conclusion

Transitioning to and maintaining a kidney-friendly diet can be challenging, but with the right strategies and support, it is entirely achievable. By addressing common challenges and leveraging community support and resources, you can navigate this journey more effectively and enjoy the numerous health benefits that come with a kidney-friendly lifestyle. Remember, you are not alone in this journey. Reach out to your community, utilize available resources, and stay committed to your health and well-being.

Chapter 24: Long-Term Maintenance
Introduction

Adopting a kidney-friendly diet is not just a short-term solution but a long-term commitment to maintaining kidney health and overall well-being. Sustaining this diet over the long term requires planning, adaptability, and a focus on making it a part of your lifestyle. This chapter provides strategies for long-term maintenance of the kidney-friendly diet and explores how to adapt the diet to different life stages and evolving health needs.

How to Sustain the Diet Long-Term

1. **Establishing Healthy Habits**:
   - **Routine and Consistency**: Develop a consistent meal planning and preparation routine. Consistency helps make the diet a natural part of your lifestyle.
   - **Daily Practices**: Incorporate daily practices such as drinking plenty of water, consuming balanced meals, and avoiding processed foods. Over time, these practices will become second nature.
2. **Continual Learning and Adaptation**:
   - **Stay Informed**: Keep up-to-date with the latest research and recommendations for kidney health and nutrition. This knowledge will help you make informed decisions and adapt your diet as needed.
   - **Experiment with Recipes**: Continually explore new recipes and cooking techniques to keep your meals exciting and varied. This helps prevent boredom and keeps you engaged with the diet.
3. **Set Realistic Goals**:

- **Short-Term Goals**: Set achievable short-term goals, such as trying a new vegetable each week or reducing sodium intake by a certain amount.
- **Long-Term Goals**: Establish long-term goals that focus on overall health and kidney function. Regularly review and adjust these goals as needed.

4. **Monitor Your Progress:**
   - **Track Health Indicators**: Keep track of key health indicators such as blood pressure, weight, and kidney function tests. Monitoring progress helps you stay motivated and make necessary adjustments.
   - **Adjust Diet Accordingly**: Based on your health indicators and any changes in your condition, adjust your diet to better meet your needs. This may involve consulting with healthcare professionals.

5. **Building a Support System:**
   - **Family and Friends**: Engage your family and friends in your dietary journey. Their support can make it easier to stay committed.
   - **Support Groups**: Join kidney health support groups, either in person or online, to share experiences, challenges, and successes with others who understand your journey.

6. **Addressing Setbacks:**
   - **Anticipate Challenges**: Recognize that setbacks are a natural part of any long-term commitment. Prepare for potential challenges, such as holidays or social gatherings, and have strategies in place to handle them.
   - **Self-Compassion**: Practice self-compassion. If you have a setback, don't be too hard on yourself. Reflect on what happened, learn from it, and refocus on your goals.

Adapting the Diet to Different Life Stages and Health Needs

1. **Adolescence:**
   - **Nutritional Requirements**: Adolescents require higher amounts of certain nutrients such as calcium and iron for growth and development. Ensure their diet includes sufficient lean proteins, dairy alternatives, and leafy greens.
   - **Engagement**: Involve adolescents in meal planning and preparation. Teaching them about healthy eating habits early on sets a foundation for lifelong health.

2. **Adulthood:**
   - **Balanced Diet**: Continue to focus on a balanced diet that includes lean proteins, whole grains, healthy fats, and plenty of fruits and vegetables.
   - **Stress and Busy Schedules**: For busy adults, meal prepping and planning are essential. Batch cooking on weekends and having healthy snacks readily available can help maintain the diet.

3. **Pregnancy:**
   - **Increased Nutritional Needs**: Pregnant women have increased nutritional needs, including folic acid, iron, calcium, and protein. Ensure these nutrients are included in the diet through kidney-friendly foods like leafy greens, legumes, and lean meats.
   - **Hydration**: Proper hydration is critical during pregnancy. Drink plenty of water and avoid high-sodium foods to prevent fluid retention and maintain kidney health.

4. **Seniors:**
   - **Digestive Health**: Seniors may experience changes in digestion and appetite. Focus on easily digestible foods and smaller, more frequent meals.
   - **Bone Health**: Ensure adequate intake of calcium and vitamin D through fortified foods or supplements to support bone health.

- **Monitoring and Adjustments**: Regularly monitor kidney function and adjust the diet based on any changes in health status. Seniors may need to reduce protein intake or manage other dietary restrictions more closely.

5. **Chronic Kidney Disease (CKD) Progression**:
   - **Stage-Specific Diet**: As CKD progresses, dietary needs change. Work closely with a dietitian to adjust protein, sodium, potassium, and phosphorus intake according to the stage of CKD.
   - **Fluid Management**: For advanced stages, fluid management becomes crucial. Monitor fluid intake and output carefully to avoid overhydration or dehydration.

Sample Long-Term Meal Plan for Different Life Stages
Adolescence: Day 1:

- **Breakfast**: Smoothie with spinach, banana, almond milk, and chia seeds
- **Lunch**: Turkey and avocado wrap with a side of carrot sticks
- **Snack**: Greek yogurt with fresh berries
- **Dinner**: Grilled chicken breast with steamed broccoli and quinoa

Adulthood: Day 1:

- **Breakfast**: Oatmeal topped with sliced banana and walnuts
- **Lunch**: Quinoa salad with chickpeas, cherry tomatoes, cucumber, and olive oil dressing
- **Snack**: Apple slices with almond butter
- **Dinner**: Baked salmon with roasted Brussels sprouts and sweet potato

Pregnancy: Day 1:

- **Breakfast**: Scrambled eggs with spinach and tomatoes
- **Lunch**: Lentil soup with a side of whole grain bread
- **Snack**: A handful of almonds and dried apricots
- **Dinner**: Roasted chicken thighs with sautéed kale and garlic, served with brown rice

Seniors: Day 1:

- **Breakfast**: Greek yogurt with granola and fresh strawberries
- **Lunch**: Vegetable stir-fry with tofu and brown rice
- **Snack**: Celery sticks with hummus
- **Dinner**: Baked cod with a side of steamed green beans and wild rice

CKD Progression: Day 1:

- **Breakfast**: Smoothie bowl with kale, pineapple, almond milk, and chia seeds
- **Lunch**: Grilled chicken Caesar salad with a light dressing
- **Snack**: Sliced bell peppers with guacamole
- **Dinner**: Turkey meatballs with spaghetti squash and marinara sauce (low sodium)

Tips for Long-Term Success

1. **Continuous Education:**
   - **Stay Updated**: Nutrition science evolves, so stay informed about the latest research and recommendations. Subscribe to reputable health newsletters and attend seminars or webinars.
   - **Educate Yourself**: Take time to understand the nutritional needs specific to your condition and life stage. Knowledge empowers you to make better choices.

2. **Flexibility and Adaptability:**
   - **Adjust as Needed**: Be willing to adapt your diet as your health needs change. Regularly review your dietary plan with healthcare professionals.
   - **Flexible Choices**: Have a list of go-to meals and snacks that can be easily adjusted based on availability and seasonality.

3. **Sustainable Habits:**
   - **Healthy Routines**: Develop daily routines that incorporate your dietary needs effortlessly. Routine helps embed these habits into your lifestyle.
   - **Mindful Eating**: Practice mindful eating to stay aware of your hunger and satiety cues. This helps prevent overeating and maintains a balanced diet.

4. **Positive Mindset:**
   - **Stay Positive**: Maintain a positive outlook on your dietary journey. Celebrate your successes and learn from challenges without self-criticism.
   - **Enjoy the Journey**: Focus on the benefits you experience, such as increased energy, better health, and improved quality of life.

Conclusion

Sustaining a kidney-friendly diet long-term is essential for maintaining kidney health and overall well-being. By establishing healthy habits, staying informed, and adapting the diet to different life stages and health needs, you can ensure the diet remains a positive and integral part of your lifestyle. Remember, this journey is about continuous improvement and maintaining a balance that supports your health. With dedication and the right strategies, you can enjoy the benefits of the kidney-friendly diet for years to come.

Chapter 25: Enhancing the Diet with Supplements

Introduction

While a well-balanced diet is the cornerstone of kidney health, supplements can provide additional support by addressing nutritional gaps and enhancing overall health. This chapter explores recommended supplements to support kidney health and provides guidance on how to safely incorporate them into your diet.

Recommended Supplements to Support Kidney Health

1. **Vitamin D:**
   - **Importance**: Vitamin D is crucial for calcium absorption and bone health. It also plays a role in immune function and inflammation reduction, which are important for kidney health.
   - **Sources**: While sunlight is a primary source of vitamin D, dietary sources include fatty fish, fortified dairy alternatives, and egg yolks. Supplements can help achieve adequate levels, especially in individuals with limited sun exposure or dietary intake.

2. **Omega-3 Fatty Acids:**
   - **Importance**: Omega-3 fatty acids, particularly EPA and DHA, have anti-inflammatory properties and can help reduce inflammation in the kidneys. They also support cardiovascular health, which is closely linked to kidney function.
   - **Sources**: Omega-3s are found in fatty fish like salmon, mackerel, and sardines. Fish oil supplements are a convenient way to ensure adequate intake, especially for those who do not consume enough fish.

3. **Coenzyme Q10 (CoQ10):**

- ◦ **Importance**: CoQ10 is an antioxidant that supports cellular energy production and protects against oxidative stress. It can help improve kidney function and reduce the progression of chronic kidney disease (CKD).
- ◦ **Sources**: CoQ10 is found in small amounts in foods like organ meats, fish, and whole grains. Supplements are often necessary to achieve therapeutic levels.

4. **B Vitamins**:

- ◦ **Importance**: B vitamins, including B6, B12, and folic acid, play vital roles in energy production, red blood cell formation, and homocysteine metabolism. High homocysteine levels are associated with increased risk of kidney disease and cardiovascular issues.
- ◦ **Sources**: B vitamins are found in a variety of foods, including lean meats, eggs, dairy alternatives, and fortified cereals. A B-complex supplement can ensure adequate intake.

5. **Magnesium**:

- ◦ **Importance**: Magnesium supports muscle and nerve function, regulates blood pressure, and helps maintain normal heart rhythm. It also plays a role in reducing the risk of kidney stones.
- ◦ **Sources**: Magnesium is found in leafy greens, nuts, seeds, and whole grains. Supplements can help individuals who have difficulty meeting their needs through diet alone.

6. **Probiotics**:

- ◦ **Importance**: Probiotics promote a healthy gut microbiome, which is essential for overall health and immune function. They can help reduce inflammation and improve nutrient absorption, benefiting kidney health.
- ◦ **Sources**: Probiotics are found in fermented foods like yogurt, kefir, sauerkraut, and kimchi. Probiotic supplements provide a concentrated dose of beneficial bacteria.

7. **Calcium**:

- ○ **Importance**: Calcium is essential for bone health and helps prevent osteoporosis, a common concern for individuals with kidney disease. It also plays a role in muscle function and blood clotting.
- ○ **Sources**: Calcium is found in dairy alternatives, leafy greens, and fortified foods. Supplements can help those who do not get enough calcium from their diet.

8. **Iron**:

- ○ **Importance**: Iron is critical for the production of hemoglobin, which carries oxygen in the blood. Anemia is common in individuals with kidney disease, making adequate iron intake essential.
- ○ **Sources**: Iron is found in red meat, poultry, fish, and fortified cereals. Iron supplements may be necessary for those with low levels.

9. **Vitamin C**:

- ○ **Importance**: Vitamin C is an antioxidant that supports immune function and helps protect against oxidative stress. It also aids in the absorption of non-heme iron from plant-based foods.
- ○ **Sources**: Vitamin C is abundant in fruits and vegetables like oranges, strawberries, bell peppers, and broccoli. Supplements can ensure adequate intake, especially during illness or stress.

10. **Alpha Lipoic Acid (ALA)**:

- ○ **Importance**: ALA is an antioxidant that helps protect cells from oxidative damage and supports metabolic health. It can benefit individuals with CKD by reducing oxidative stress.
- ○ **Sources**: ALA is found in small amounts in foods like spinach, broccoli, and organ meats. Supplements are often used to achieve therapeutic benefits.

How to Safely Incorporate Supplements into the Diet

1. **Consult with Healthcare Professionals:**
   - **Medical Advice:** Always consult with your healthcare provider or a registered dietitian before starting any new supplement. They can assess your individual needs, current medications, and potential interactions.
   - **Monitoring:** Regular monitoring of kidney function and overall health is essential to ensure that supplements are providing the intended benefits and not causing harm.
2. **Start with the Basics:**
   - **Essential Supplements:** Begin with the most essential supplements based on your specific health needs. Common starting points include vitamin D, omega-3 fatty acids, and a B-complex vitamin.
   - **Gradual Introduction:** Introduce one supplement at a time to monitor its effects and ensure it is well-tolerated.
3. **Quality and Dosage:**
   - **Reputable Brands:** Choose high-quality supplements from reputable brands that are third-party tested for purity and potency.
   - **Correct Dosage:** Follow the recommended dosage provided by your healthcare provider. More is not always better, and excessive intake of certain supplements can be harmful.
4. **Timing and Absorption:**
   - **With Meals:** Some supplements, such as fat-soluble vitamins (A, D, E, K) and CoQ10, are better absorbed when taken with meals that contain fat.
   - **Split Doses:** For better absorption and to reduce potential side effects, split the daily dose of certain supplements, such as magnesium or probiotics, into smaller doses taken throughout the day.

5. **Be Aware of Interactions:**
  - **Medication Interactions**: Certain supplements can interact with medications. For example, vitamin K can interfere with blood thinners, and high doses of calcium can affect the absorption of certain medications.
  - **Nutrient Interactions**: Some nutrients compete for absorption. For example, calcium can interfere with iron absorption, so it may be best to take them at different times.
6. **Monitor for Side Effects:**
  - **Adverse Reactions**: Be vigilant for any adverse reactions or side effects when starting a new supplement. Common side effects can include gastrointestinal discomfort, headaches, or allergic reactions.
  - **Adjust as Needed**: If side effects occur, consult your healthcare provider to adjust the dosage or discontinue the supplement.

Sample Supplement Routine for Kidney Health
Morning:

- **Vitamin D**: 1000-2000 IU with breakfast
- **Omega-3 Fatty Acids**: 1000 mg with breakfast
- **B-Complex Vitamin**: 1 tablet with breakfast
- **Probiotic**: 1 capsule before breakfast

Afternoon:

- **Magnesium**: 250-400 mg with lunch
- **Vitamin C**: 500 mg with lunch

Evening:

- **CoQ10**: 100 mg with dinner

- **Calcium**: 500 mg with dinner

As Needed:

- **Iron**: Based on individual needs and blood test results
- **Alpha Lipoic Acid**: 300 mg with lunch or dinner

Conclusion

Incorporating supplements into your kidney-friendly diet can provide additional support for maintaining optimal kidney health and overall well-being. However, it is essential to approach supplementation with caution and under the guidance of healthcare professionals. By choosing the right supplements, following proper dosages, and monitoring your health, you can enhance the benefits of your diet and support your long-term health goals. Remember, supplements are intended to complement, not replace, a balanced diet and healthy lifestyle.

Chapter 26: Exercise and Kidney Health

Introduction

Physical activity plays a crucial role in maintaining overall health and supporting kidney function. Regular exercise can help manage risk factors associated with kidney disease, such as high blood pressure, obesity, and diabetes, while also promoting cardiovascular health and improving mental well-being. This chapter explores the role of physical activity in supporting kidney function and provides recommended exercises and routines tailored to different fitness levels and health conditions.

Role of Physical Activity in Supporting Kidney Function

1. **Improving Cardiovascular Health**:
   - **Enhanced Blood Flow**: Regular exercise improves blood circulation, which enhances oxygen and nutrient delivery to the kidneys. This supports their function and helps maintain overall kidney health.
   - **Lowering Blood Pressure**: Physical activity helps lower blood pressure, reducing the strain on the kidneys and decreasing the risk of hypertension, a leading cause of kidney disease.

2. **Managing Weight**:
   - **Weight Loss and Maintenance**: Exercise aids in weight loss and helps maintain a healthy weight. Obesity is a significant risk factor for kidney disease, so maintaining a healthy weight reduces this risk.
   - **Fat Reduction**: Regular physical activity helps reduce visceral fat, the type of fat that surrounds internal organs,

which can improve kidney function and reduce inflammation.

3. **Controlling Blood Sugar Levels:**
   - **Improved Insulin Sensitivity**: Exercise enhances insulin sensitivity, helping to regulate blood sugar levels. This is particularly important for individuals with diabetes, as uncontrolled diabetes can lead to kidney damage.
   - **Lower Blood Sugar**: Regular physical activity helps lower blood sugar levels, reducing the risk of developing diabetic nephropathy, a common complication of diabetes affecting the kidneys.

4. **Reducing Inflammation:**
   - **Anti-Inflammatory Effects**: Exercise has anti-inflammatory effects, which can help reduce chronic inflammation that contributes to kidney damage.
   - **Enhanced Immune Function**: Regular physical activity supports a healthy immune system, which can help protect the kidneys from infections and other inflammatory conditions.

5. **Enhancing Mental Health:**
   - **Stress Reduction**: Physical activity reduces stress levels and promotes mental well-being. Stress can negatively impact kidney health, so managing stress through exercise is beneficial.
   - **Improved Mood**: Exercise releases endorphins, which improve mood and provide a sense of well-being. This can motivate individuals to adhere to a kidney-friendly diet and lifestyle.

Recommended Exercises and Routines

1. **Aerobic Exercise:**

- ◦ **Benefits**: Aerobic exercise improves cardiovascular health, aids in weight loss, and enhances overall endurance.
  - ◦ **Examples**: Walking, jogging, cycling, swimming, dancing, and using cardio machines like treadmills and ellipticals.
  - ◦ **Routine**: Aim for at least 150 minutes of moderate-intensity aerobic exercise per week or 75 minutes of vigorous-intensity exercise, spread across several days.

2. **Strength Training**:
   - ◦ **Benefits**: Strength training builds muscle mass, increases metabolism, and improves bone density. It also helps with weight management and overall physical function.
   - ◦ **Examples**: Weight lifting, resistance band exercises, body-weight exercises (such as squats, lunges, push-ups), and using weight machines.
   - ◦ **Routine**: Incorporate strength training exercises at least two days per week, focusing on all major muscle groups.

3. **Flexibility and Balance Exercises**:
   - ◦ **Benefits**: Flexibility exercises improve range of motion, reduce the risk of injury, and enhance overall physical performance. Balance exercises help prevent falls and improve stability.
   - ◦ **Examples**: Stretching routines, yoga, Pilates, tai chi, and balance drills (such as standing on one foot).
   - ◦ **Routine**: Include flexibility and balance exercises 2-3 times per week, ideally after aerobic or strength training sessions.

4. **Low-Impact Exercises**:
   - ◦ **Benefits**: Low-impact exercises are gentler on the joints and suitable for individuals with joint pain or mobility issues.
   - ◦ **Examples**: Swimming, water aerobics, walking, cycling, and elliptical training.
   - ◦ **Routine**: Aim for at least 30 minutes of low-impact exercise most days of the week, adjusting intensity based on fitness level and comfort.

5. **High-Intensity Interval Training (HIIT):**
    - **Benefits**: HIIT involves short bursts of intense exercise followed by rest or low-intensity exercise. It improves cardiovascular fitness, burns calories efficiently, and enhances metabolic health.
    - **Examples**: Sprint intervals, circuit training, and high-intensity bodyweight exercises.
    - **Routine**: Incorporate HIIT workouts 1-2 times per week, with sessions lasting 20-30 minutes.

Sample Exercise Routine for Kidney Health
Beginner Routine:

- **Monday:**
    - 30-minute brisk walk
    - 10 minutes of stretching
- **Wednesday:**
    - 20 minutes of cycling
    - 10 minutes of bodyweight exercises (squats, lunges, push-ups)
- **Friday:**
    - 30-minute water aerobics
    - 10 minutes of balance exercises (standing on one foot, heel-to-toe walk)

Intermediate Routine:

- **Monday:**
    - 30-minute jog
    - 15 minutes of strength training (dumbbells or resistance bands)
- **Wednesday:**
    - 30-minute elliptical session

- ° 10 minutes of yoga or stretching
- **Friday:**
    - ° 20-minute HIIT workout (sprints, jumping jacks, burpees)
    - ° 10 minutes of core exercises (planks, bicycle crunches)
- **Saturday:**
    - ° 45-minute hike or outdoor activity
    - ° 10 minutes of stretching

Advanced Routine:

- **Monday:**
    - ° 40-minute run
    - ° 20 minutes of strength training (free weights or machines)
- **Wednesday:**
    - ° 30-minute swim
    - ° 15 minutes of Pilates
- **Friday:**
    - ° 30-minute HIIT workout (circuit training with various exercises)
    - ° 10 minutes of flexibility exercises
- **Saturday:**
    - ° 60-minute bike ride or long-distance run
    - ° 15 minutes of yoga

Tips for Safe and Effective Exercise

1. **Consult with Healthcare Providers:**
    - ° **Medical Clearance:** Before starting a new exercise routine, consult with your healthcare provider, especially if you have chronic kidney disease or other health conditions.
    - ° **Personalized Advice:** Seek personalized advice from a healthcare provider or fitness professional to create a safe and effective exercise plan.

2. **Start Slowly**:
    - **Gradual Progression**: Begin with low-intensity exercises and gradually increase the intensity and duration as your fitness level improves.
    - **Listen to Your Body**: Pay attention to how your body responds to exercise. If you experience pain, dizziness, or excessive fatigue, stop exercising and consult your healthcare provider.
3. **Stay Hydrated**:
    - **Proper Hydration**: Drink water before, during, and after exercise to stay hydrated. Proper hydration supports kidney function and overall performance.
    - **Avoid Overhydration**: Balance fluid intake to avoid overhydration, which can strain the kidneys.
4. **Warm-Up and Cool-Down**:
    - **Warm-Up**: Begin each exercise session with a warm-up to prepare your muscles and cardiovascular system. A 5-10 minute warm-up of light aerobic activity and dynamic stretching is recommended.
    - **Cool-Down**: End each session with a cool-down to gradually reduce heart rate and stretch muscles. This helps prevent injury and aids recovery.
5. **Consistency and Variety**:
    - **Regular Exercise**: Aim for consistency in your exercise routine. Regular physical activity provides the most health benefits.
    - **Variety**: Incorporate a variety of exercises to work different muscle groups and prevent boredom. Mixing up your routine can also improve overall fitness.

Conclusion

Exercise is a vital component of maintaining kidney health and overall well-being. Regular physical activity supports cardiovascular health, weight management, blood sugar control, and reduces inflammation, all of which are crucial for optimal kidney function. By incorporating a balanced exercise routine that includes aerobic, strength, flexibility, and balance exercises, you can enhance your health and quality of life. Remember to consult with healthcare professionals, start slowly, and listen to your body to ensure safe and effective exercise. With commitment and consistency, you can enjoy the numerous benefits that regular physical activity brings to your kidney health and overall well-being.

Chapter 27: Final Thoughts and Encouragement
Summary of Key Points

As we come to the conclusion of "10X: The Kidney Friendly Diet," let's take a moment to recap the essential elements we've covered throughout this journey. This book has provided comprehensive guidance on how to support and enhance kidney health through dietary and lifestyle changes. Here are the key points:

1. **Understanding Kidney Health**:
   - The kidneys play a vital role in filtering waste and maintaining overall body balance.
   - Protecting kidney health involves managing factors like blood pressure, blood sugar, and hydration.

2. **Dietary Foundations**:
   - A kidney-friendly diet emphasizes whole foods, lean proteins, healthy fats, and low sodium intake.
   - Avoiding processed foods, sugars, and seed oils is crucial for reducing the burden on the kidneys.

3. **Hydration**:
   - Proper hydration with alkaline and reverse osmosis water supports kidney function and overall health.
   - Avoid sugary drinks and sodas to prevent additional strain on the kidneys.

4. **Nutrient-Rich Foods**:
   - Focus on nutrient-dense foods like leafy greens, berries, fatty fish, nuts, and seeds.
   - Incorporate foods that are low in potassium and phosphorus if necessary, based on individual kidney health.

5. **Supplements**:

- ◦ Certain supplements, such as vitamin D, omega-3 fatty acids, and CoQ10, can provide additional support for kidney health.
- ◦ Always consult with healthcare professionals before starting any new supplements.

6. **Exercise:**
- ◦ Regular physical activity supports cardiovascular health, weight management, and overall well-being.
- ◦ Aim for a balanced exercise routine that includes aerobic, strength, flexibility, and balance exercises.

7. **Monitoring and Adjustments:**
- ◦ Regular check-ups and monitoring of kidney function are essential for making necessary dietary adjustments.
- ◦ Use tools like food diaries and health apps to track progress and stay informed.

8. **Coping with Challenges:**
- ◦ Address common challenges such as cravings, social situations, and time management with practical strategies.
- ◦ Build a support system through family, friends, and community resources.

9. **Long-Term Maintenance:**
- ◦ Establish healthy habits, stay informed, and adapt the diet to different life stages and health needs.
- ◦ Consistency and flexibility are key to maintaining the diet long-term.

10. **Community and Resources:**
- ◦ Leverage community support and educational resources to stay motivated and informed.
- ◦ Engage with support groups and healthcare professionals for ongoing guidance.

Encouragement and Motivation for Continuing the Diet

Embarking on a kidney-friendly diet is a significant and commendable commitment to your health. It's natural to encounter challenges along the way, but it's important to remember why you started and the benefits you're working towards. Here are some words of encouragement to help you stay motivated:

1. **Celebrate Your Progress**:
   - Every small step you take towards a healthier diet is a victory. Celebrate your progress, whether it's a week of healthy eating, a successful workout, or improved lab results.
   - Acknowledge the positive changes you feel, such as increased energy, better mood, and enhanced well-being.

2. **Stay Focused on the Benefits**:
   - Keep in mind the long-term benefits of the kidney-friendly diet, including better kidney function, reduced risk of chronic diseases, and improved overall health.
   - Visualize your health goals and remind yourself of the reasons why you embarked on this journey.

3. **Embrace Flexibility and Adaptability**:
   - Life is dynamic, and so are your health needs. Be flexible and willing to adapt your diet and lifestyle as needed.
   - Remember that perfection is not the goal; consistency and dedication are what matter most.

4. **Build a Supportive Environment**:
   - Surround yourself with supportive friends, family, and community members who understand and respect your dietary choices.
   - Seek out online communities, support groups, and educational resources to stay connected and motivated.

5. **Prioritize Self-Care**:
   - Taking care of your mental and emotional health is just as important as physical health. Practice self-compassion

and prioritize self-care activities that bring you joy and relaxation.

- Manage stress through healthy outlets like exercise, meditation, hobbies, and social connections.

6. **Learn and Grow:**

- Continue to educate yourself about kidney health and nutrition. Staying informed empowers you to make the best choices for your health.
- Experiment with new recipes and foods to keep your diet interesting and enjoyable.

Final Words from the Author

As the author of "10X: The Kidney Friendly Diet," I want to express my heartfelt gratitude for joining me on this journey. Writing this book has been a labor of love, inspired by my own experiences and the desire to help others achieve better kidney health and overall well-being.

Commitment and perseverance are the cornerstones of any successful health journey. The road to better health is not always easy, but it is incredibly rewarding. By making informed choices and staying dedicated to your goals, you are taking control of your health and future.

Remember, you are not alone in this journey. There is a community of individuals and professionals ready to support you every step of the way. Reach out, ask for help, and share your experiences. Together, we can achieve great things.

Stay committed to your health, embrace the changes, and persevere through the challenges. Your efforts will pay off, and you will enjoy the many benefits of a kidney-friendly diet and lifestyle. Here's to your health, happiness, and longevity.

Thank you for trusting me as your guide on this journey. Wishing you all the best on your path to optimal kidney health and beyond.

With gratitude and encouragement,
Matthew Petchinsky

Conclusion

"10X: The Kidney Friendly Diet" has provided you with the tools, knowledge, and support needed to embark on a journey towards better kidney health. By following the guidelines and embracing the principles outlined in this book, you can achieve and maintain optimal kidney function and overall well-being.

Stay committed, stay informed, and stay motivated. Your health is worth every effort.

Message from the Author:

I hope you enjoyed this book, I love astrology and knew there was not a book such as this out on the shelf. I love metaphysical items as well. Please check out my other books:

-Life of Government Benefits

-My life of Hell

-My life with Hydrocephalus

-Red Sky

-World Domination:Woman's rule

-World Domination:Woman's Rule 2: The War

-Life and Banishment of Apophis: book 1

-The Kidney Friendly Diet

-The Ultimate Hemp Cookbook

-Creating a Dispensary(legally)

-Cleanliness throughout life: the importance of showering from childhood to adulthood.

-Strong Roots: The Risks of Overcoddling children

-Hemp Horoscopes: Cosmic Insights and Earthly Healing

- Celestial Hemp Navigating the Zodiac: Through the Green Cosmos

-Astrological Hemp: Aligning The Stars with Earth's Ancient Herb

-The Astrological Guide to Hemp: Stars, Signs, and Sacred Leaves

-Green Growth: Innovative Marketing Strategies for your Hemp Products and Dispensary

-Cosmic Cannabis

-Astrological Munchies

-Henry The Hemp

-Zodiacal Roots: The Astrological Soul Of Hemp

- **Green Constellations: Intersection of Hemp and Zodiac**

-Hemp in The Houses: An astrological Adventure Through The Cannabis Galaxy

-Galactic Ganja Guide

Heavenly Hemp

Zodiac Leaves

Doctor Who Astrology

Cannastrology

Stellar Satvias and Cosmic Indicas

Celestial Cannabis: A Zodiac Journey

AstroHerbology: The Sky and The Soil: Volume 1

AstroHerbology:Celestial Cannabis:Volume 2

Cosmic Cannabis Cultivation

The Starry Guide to Herbal Harmony: Volume 1

The Starry Guide to Herbal Harmony: Cannabis Universe: Volume 2

Yugioh Astrology: Astrological Guide to Deck, Duels and more

Nightmare Mansion: Echoes of The Abyss

Nightmare Mansion 2: Legacy of Shadows

Nightmare Mansion 3: Shadows of the Forgotten

Nightmare Mansion 4: Echoes of the Damned

The Life and Banishment of Apophis: Book 2

Nightmare Mansion: Halls of Despair

Healing with Herb: Cannabis and Hydrocephalus

Planetary Pot: Aligning with Astrological Herbs: Volume 1

Fast Track to Freedom: 30 Days to Financial Independence Using AI, Assets, and Agile Hustles

Cosmic Hemp Pathways

How to Become Financially Free in 30 Days: 10,000 Paths to Prosperity

Zodiacal Herbage: Astrological Insights: Volume 1

Nightmare Mansion: Whispers in the Walls
The Daleks Invade Atlantis
Henry the hemp and Hydrocephalus

Check out my Virtual dispensary for all your hemp needs: https://shift.store/sg1fan23477/retail

If you want solar for your home go here: https://www.harborsolar.live/apophisenterprises/

Instagrams:
@apophis_enterprises,
@hempkingdom2024,
@apophisbookemporium,
@apophisfashion,
@apophisscardshop
Twitter: @apophisenterpr1,
Tiktok:@apophisenterprise
Youtube: @sg1fan23477
Podcast:Apophis Chat Zone: https://open.spotify.com/show/5zXbrCLEV2xzCp8ybrfHsk?si=fb4d4fdbdce44dec

Newsletter: https://apophiss-newsletter-27c897.beehiiv.com/
Shirt shop: www.bonfire.com/store/apophis-shirt-emporium/